Many significant r̶_____
California over th_____
all have in comm_____
sionate voice of Jeff Baugh telling the story from high
above. As I think about those stories it's Jeff's voice I hear
narrating them in my head much like the way Vin Scully
would call a key ninth inning of a Dodgers playoff game.
This book accomplishes in print what Jeff has done for so
many on the radio.

—KEN CHARLES, Program Director, KNX 1070 News Radio

Stick With Us and We'll Get You There provides a unique and
creative approach to facing life's challenges. So many of us
spend so much of our lives "on the road". Driving has many
meanings both pragmatically and psychologically. Walker
Baron and Baugh, in their different but compatible perspectives, employing freeway driving and road metaphors, touch
the life experiences of so many individuals. Their book will
certainly provide insight into life's challenges.

—JUDITH KAUFMAN, Ph.D., ABPP Professor and
Director of School Psychology
Training-Fairleigh Dickinson University

The Southern California complex freeway system is something to behold, maybe the best in the world in its connec-
tive tissue with communities. The only problem is that it
doesn't work so well for much of the time. When the traffic
jam stops us in our tracks, we wonder why. Jeff and Mary
rip the curtain back to tell us the story in this book that is
powerful for the commuter, the student, and politician.
Get out of your car and buy this book!

—DON BARRETT, founder of LA Radio People
and LARadio.com

Stick With Us And We'll Get You There is creative, imaginative, resourceful and intriguing as we join Los Angles and life roadway traffic. Imagine flying in an airplane to discover self-help skills. This book helps us stay alert to maintain good mental and emotional health. I've already used the concept of Botts Dots with my clients.

—HEATHER HALPERIN, LCSW-recipient of the
National Association of Social Workers'
Life Time Achievement Award

This is a captivating, courageous and insanely creative book. It juxtaposes perspectives that shed light on deeper meanings of familiar scenes.

—DR. MELISSA INDERA SINGH, LCSW

STICK WITH US
AND WE'LL
GET YOU THERE

OTHER WORKS PUBLISHED BY STEEL CUT PRESS:

But This Is Different

Of Little Faith

Hoarding Lies, Keeping Secrets

Leaning On God: Sermons of Rabbi Carole L. Meyers

Happy Birthday
Jeff
— David
+
Andrea
Allen
10/2018

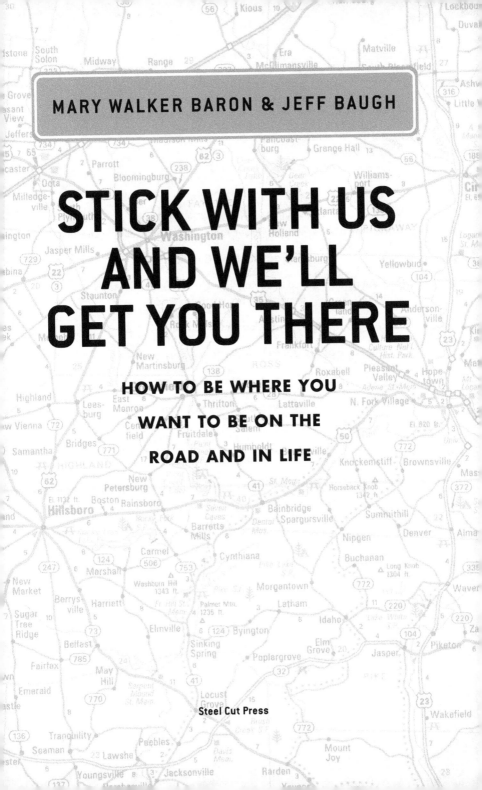

MARY WALKER BARON & JEFF BAUGH

STICK WITH US AND WE'LL GET YOU THERE

HOW TO BE WHERE YOU WANT TO BE ON THE WANT TO BE ON THE ROAD AND IN LIFE

Steel Cut Press

Stick With Us And We'll Get You There:
How To Be Where You Want To Be On The Road And In Life

@2018 by Steel Cut Press

Photography by Jeff Baugh and David G. Hall.

Book Design by Neuwirth & Associates, Inc.

Cover Concept by Jesse Leffler

Cover Design by Tim Green

ISBNs:

Print - 978-1-936380-08-4 and 1-936380-08-0
Kindle - 978-1-936380-09-1 and 1-936380-09-9
EPUB - 978-1-936380-10-7 and 1-936380-10-2

LCCN: 2016958706

Steel Cut Press
www.SteelCutPress.com

FROM JEFF: I dedicate this book with love and respect to Mildred, Robin and Brian. If there was anyone who needed a way or two around a problem that I drove into a long time ago I was that person. I'm better now, much better. I also dedicate it to "my gift from God" Mary Walker.

FROM MARY: I dedicate this book with love and respect to Leslie Bergson, Jesse, Mike, Charles and Claire Leffler and, of course, Jeff Baugh for sticking with me.

There's one other person we must thank—Dr. Loretta Howitt. Without Dr. Howitt Jeff would never have heard of Mary. Here's what happened. Mary served a two-year term as president of her synagogue. Part of her responsibilities was to write a monthly article for the synagogue newsletter. Dr. Howitt thought that Jeff should read one particular article written just before the Jewish New Year. She sent him a copy. The unopened envelope rattled around radio station KFWB 980 AM for a while and almost got thrown away. Finally someone got it to Jeff. He read it. That's how and when the friendship started.

Thank you, Loretta. Without you this book would not exist.

You can find that article in the back of the book if you want to take a look at it.

Here's what we've got for you:

WHO WE ARE AND WHY YOU SHOULD STICK WITH US

"To be a credible, successful airborne reporter, you only need to live by a few rules. Know your audience and what they're probably doing while you're speaking to them. The television audience is for the most part at home or work. The radio listener is probably driving. Most of all don't 'report.' Just talk. And finally: Always be looking at what you're talking about!"

—JEFF BAUGH

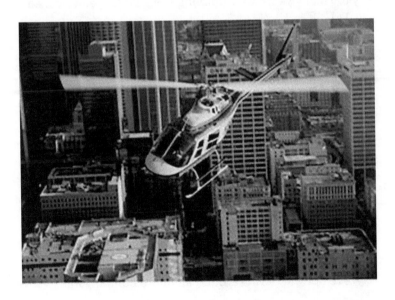

ERE'S THE FIRST THING you should know about the authors of this book. We've been around the block a few times. It wasn't always the same block and more often than not it wasn't even a block we wanted to go around. We've occasionally gone in the wrong direction and wandered pointlessly trying to find our way back to where we started. We've made stupid decisions. We've wasted time and effort and money. Many stages of our journeys initially lacked proper planning. Okay. In all honesty they weren't planned at all. We knew we were looking for something. We just didn't know what it was or how to find it. When we finally realized what it was, we still didn't know how to get there. We spent way too many years just bumbling along often feeling lost and a little foolish.

Does any of this sound familiar? Yeah. That's what we thought. You've been there. You've done that. And still your life just seems to lack direction.

We can help you get to where you want to go.

You just need a tour guide. We could all use one or two from time to time. So who better to guide you to your destinations than a couple of people who know the roads like the backs of their hands? You want a tour guide who knows the territory and who won't get lost. We are the tour guides you need. We really can help you and we really want to do just that.

So listen up!

We're not wandering around anymore bumping into every

hazard the journey can offer. We've figured out a few things. In fact, we've spent the last few decades each in our own way helping people get to where they want to go.

Jeff's voice is one of the best known in Los Angeles. People listen to him every morning and every evening as he tells them how to navigate the Los Angeles freeway systems getting to where they want to go.

Jeff is a native New Yorker who grew up in the Flatbush and Coney Island sections of Brooklyn. He went to high school in the suburbs of the North Shore of Long Island. After graduation he served in the United States Marine Corps for seven years. He returned to civilian life able to admit he ruined a wonderful marriage and lost a precious family. Reeling from that self-inflicted catastrophe, he held down

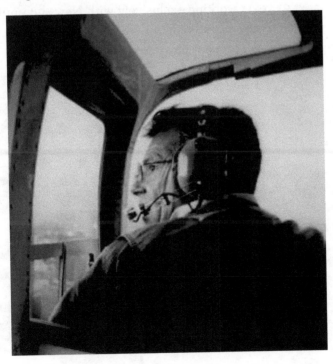

unfulfilling jobs in automobile retail and wholesale trade.

In the early 1970s an underground movement started in New York City that was eventually called Rent or Loft parties. These parties became dance clubs with disc jockeys flawlessly spinning and mixing records. This type of DJ music kept the dance floors packed. Jeff was one of those early movement DJs. Later in that decade he moved to Los Angeles and continued working in clubs and promoting the records he played.

Late in the 1980s a friend mentored Jeff into a broadcasting school and the resulting internships. When a position at Metro Traffic in Los Angeles opened, Jeff applied. He was assigned to the all-news radio station KFWB News 98 and quickly moved from the studio to airborne reporter. He spent the next 21 years working exclusively with News 98 until a corporate change moved him to KNX 1070 News Radio Los Angeles. His most recent move is to KFI AM 640 where as

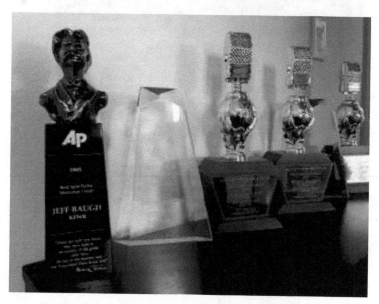

the KFI In The Sky he continues flying above the traffic helping people get through it. Jeff has received awards from the State of California, the City of Los Angeles and most of its neighboring cities and many private agencies. The Associated Press and the Radio and Television News Association have recognized him for excellence in broadcasting.

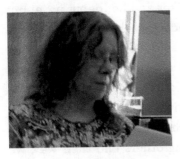

Mary was born in the Arizona State Prison where her grandfather, A. G. Walker, served as warden. Her father was a cattle rancher and Mary grew up on two different, remote, Arizona ranches. In that isolated childhood, Mary developed passions for both reading stories and writing them.

Mary received a scholarship to attend Arizona State University where for three years she spent more time in the theatre than in the classroom. Finally she embraced the 'Tune In, Turn On, Drop Out' mantra of the sixties and took a train to New York City with no plan for income or residence. She was able to locate another ASU expatriate and together they went from bad to worse. During that descent Mary sang folk songs in Greenwich Village and took on temporary office jobs. Finally she and her friend fled the city, each going their separate way.

Eventually Mary finished her undergraduate degree and later earned two Masters Degrees—one in social work from the University of Southern California and one in Jewish Communal Service from Hebrew Union College. During her graduate studies Mary realized she had inherited her grandfather's passion for social justice and social reform. As a licensed clinical social worker, she has devoted her clinical career to indigent, homeless, and severely mentally ill adults and children. Mary has written six screenplays. Her articles have appeared in both local and national newspapers and magazines. Her novels <u>Contrary Creek</u> written in collaboration with her brother Tom Walker and her debut novel <u>But This Is Different</u> continue to receive high praise. She is currently a member of the University of Southern California's Suzanne Dworak-Peck School of Social Work faculty and maintains a private therapy practice.

From our decades of wandering, we know where we want to be and we know how to get there.

From our decades of helping others find their way, we know we can help you, too.

Just stick with us and we'll get you there.

WHY WE WROTE THIS BOOK AND WHY YOU NEED TO READ IT

EVERAL YEARS AGO WE realized that what we do is almost identical. We just do it in different ways. One of us flies above the fray trying to help people get through it and the other stays on the ground doing pretty much the same thing. Essentially we are tour guides who have stumbled around finding our own paths sometimes successfully and other times disastrously but always coming back to share what we learned.

True to our often haphazard approach we one day slapped our foreheads and wondered rhetorically why not write a book. However, we gradually started taking our own advice and decided to really do it. And here it is.

We understand that you might be wondering what to do with this book now that you have it. We hope you will use it as a tool. Start at the beginning and work your way to the end or start at the end and work your way to the beginning. Choose whatever pages or sections you find interesting and read them. Skip through it in any way you wish. Write in it. In fact, there are places set aside for writing. Here's one right now. Go ahead. Write something just to prove to yourself that you can. Can't think of anything to say? Write that down. Write down your grocery list or your list of chores you want to get done before bedtime. It doesn't matter what you write. It's your book, after all. What's important is that you start right now using these pages as your personal tool.

....

....

....

....

You did it! Thank you. Now you're ready to really use this book in the way we had hoped you would. Mark it up. Dog-ear the pages. Carry it with you. Destroy it with use. You can always buy another copy to destroy with more use. That is what we hope you will do with it. What we hope you do not do is lay it down and forget about it because after all is said and done we want you to get to where you want to go both on the road and in life.

In our table of contents we listed what we've got in store for you in this book. If you glanced at that page you might have noticed that we devoted a lot of space to major 'events' impacting the flow of life and traffic in the Los Angeles free-way systems. We get it that not everyone reading this book lives in Southern California. Don't forget, though, that Los Angeles practically invented freeway traffic jams and car chases and four-level interchanges. Also keep in mind that these are the roads we know best. We've been flying over them and driving on them for decades.

We all go from one place to another and we all run into

barriers and hurdles and mishaps while we journey. It's called living. It doesn't matter that you may not know exactly what the exchange from The 110 to The 105 looks like or that it even exists. You've got your own roads to travel and we're just trying to help you get there.

We chose ten of what we consider to be major Los Angeles freeway events. We describe each event. Some of them happened years ago and others are fairly recent but all changed lives and landscapes. We want you to understand the significance of each event and its impact on people's lives. So we tell you about it. We call this section *'Listen Up! Here it is!'*

We next invite you to experience the event through Jeff's eyes. From the air he sees the whole picture. He sees what happened, what's being done about it, and how drivers can avoid getting stuck in the middle of it. He frequently receives awards for his reporting as well as for his guidance. We want to you see what Jeff saw and we want you to also experience the wisdom he shares with his listeners. We call this section *"In The Air With Jeff!"*.

His reporting and his wisdom bring us to the third part of our 'major freeway events' section. Remember that we told you we essentially do the same thing—one in the air and one on the ground? In the third section of the freeway events we combine both of our worlds.

We could probably have done nothing more with this book than tell you about the 'events' because the base reality is that we all seem to really like hearing about traffic accidents or train wrecks or seem to really need to slow down to gawk at them and some folks would have thought we'd done enough by describing the events. The evening news has enough 'looky loo' reporting to satisfy those very human curiosities. Remember that we're writing this book to help you get to where you want to go on the road and in life and not to give you one more excuse to not get there at all.

We call our third section of the events *"On The Ground With Mary!"*. This is the 'so what' component to all of this. In this section we expand the actual freeway event into an opportunity for personal learning and growth. These opportunities as presented are metaphorical in nature and designed to help us make meaning from tragedy or potential tragedy.

We believe that there has to be something we can learn from these major events and this section of our book is where the learning happens. This is not only a book about navigating Southern California traffic snarls but about navigating life snarls. We're not engineers. We're not even going to try and tell you how to keep a crane from falling across all lanes of a major freeway. We have no idea how to do that. And after all these years there's little point in reminding you that sometimes going over Laurel Canyon will get you to the Valley so you can avoid all of the snarled, stopped Hollywood Freeway. There's even less point in doing that if you live nowhere near Southern California. What we can do, though, is identify what we thought made the day more difficult for the people trying to get from one place to another. In the case of the crane, for example, it wasn't that the freeway was closed in both directions. This book is not about getting around blocked freeways. It's about staying focused and being flexible and realizing your dreams. It's about letting go of old 'stuff' we no longer need so we can get the new 'stuff' so essential to getting to where we want to be. It just so happens that we get you to the learning by connecting life challenges to freeway challenges.

We draw parallels based on the event because we can learn from each and every one if those freeway events. It's the learning that matters.

Trust us. We know that we learn as we go. We learn from our mistakes and our tragedies. We also learn from the tragedies and mistakes of others without casting blame and without unnecessary regret. The main thing is that we keep learning and finding better ways to get to where we want to go.

That might sound confusing but we promise that if you stick with us we'll help you make sense of it all.

LOS ANGELES FREEWAYS
ARE A LOT LIKE LIFE

ASIDE FROM THE OBVIOUS reasons that Jeff flies over them and Mary drives them, the Los Angeles freeway system would nevertheless have been used as the central metaphor for this book. It occupies a special place on the cultural landscape of this country and has been used metaphorically in essays and novels and movies.

Los Angeles with its almost four million residents is one of the three most populous cities in this country. New York City has over eight million residents and Chicago has almost three million residents. New York City and Chicago both have famously efficient public transportation systems. For decades Los Angeles had little if any efficient form of public transportation. True, in the early to the middle of the Twentieth Century, Los Angeles did have its Red Car streetcar line going from Pasadena to downtown Los Angeles to Santa Monica to Long Beach and connecting five counties but that system went the way of political intrigue and broken dreams.

Speaking of broken dreams, let's not underestimate the impact the movie industry had and continues to have on the cultural landscape of the nation and especially of Southern California. People flocked to Hollywood to claim their place on the cutting room floor. Everything about the place seemed so romantic. The country had a love affair with movies, with automobiles, and with Southern California because that's where the magic happened. And that's where the magic continues to happen. The award winning motion picture "La La Land" begins at the interchange of the 110 and 105 freeways.

During the 1930s and the 1940s the population of Southern California increased almost at the same pace that the price of automobiles decreased leaving Southern California desperately in need of some system to move people from one place to another. By the late 1930s traffic congestion was so bad the economy of Southern California began to suffer. In 1940 drivers began to use the Arroyo Seco Parkway to drive from Pasadena to downtown Los Angeles and back. The Arroyo Seco Parkway, later known as the Pasadena Freeway, was the first true urban freeway. The success of this first freeway paved the way for the current freeway system.

By 1947, the California Department of Public Works (Caltrans) began construction on the freeway system. The fascination with this web of concrete and asphalt continues to this day. Freeway construction also continues. So all too often does the congestion.

From its beginning the freeway system of Los Angeles has captured the imagination. Often the words "Los Angeles" and "freeway system" seem irrevocably connected. If we judged the freeway system by its place in our collective imagination we would have to determine that it was transportation perfection. Not so. According to the Federal Highway Administration, of the 36 largest metro areas Los Angeles ranks last in terms of freeway lane miles per resident. This unfortunate statistic is what keeps Jeff busy and you will see as our metaphor develops it's also what keeps Mary busy.

Although Los Angeles seems to be the epicenter of the freeway fascination it must be noted that commutes get longer and longer. Commuters traveling these freeways put in more miles than most Americans. They also spend more time stuck in traffic than most Americans. The Los Angeles freeway system must now include all of Los Angeles County (with its population of about ten million), Santa Barbara County, Ventura County, Orange County, San Diego County and the largest county in square miles in the country, San Bernardino County. That's a lot of cars and congestion and accidents.

Yet in spite of all of this, Los Angeles and its freeway system seem to captivate imagination in music, in movies, in books and in poetry and plays. To understand the City of Angeles, author Joan Didion once wrote that one needed to immerse oneself in the freeway experience. In her 1970 novel "Play It As It Lays" she shows Southern California buffeted by ". . . the weather of catastrophe, of apocalypse but grounded by its highways." The main character in the novel, Maria Wyeth, copes with personal tragedy by driving the freeway. Her car and the freeways upon which she drove, in the metaphor created by Joan Didion, allowed Maria Wyeth to carry on to the novel's conclusion.

Our metaphorical freeways can become our escape or our anchor. They can provide safe passage. They can stimulate order in increasingly chaotic lives. The architectural historian Reyner Banham's 1971 "four ecologies" looked at the way people who live in Los Angeles relate to the beach, the flatlands, the foothills and the freeways. He wrote that the Los

Angeles freeways were ". . . not a limbo of existential angst, but the place where they (commuters) spend the two calmest and most rewarding hours of their daily lives."

The daily experiences of many Southern California commuters would disprove Banham's vision of calm. Nevertheless, he did create a compelling metaphor. The Los Angeles freeway system has also been used metaphorically for 'instant gratification'. Hop on any freeway and you can be anywhere you want to be in a matter of minutes—the ocean, the mountains or the desert. Of course, Jeff on a daily basis can attest to the fallacy of that belief. Metaphorically we can skip our cares and responsibilities and just 'go to the beach'. Come to think of it, many compelling metaphors can be easily disproven. Getting stuck in traffic does not lend itself to instant gratification and fleeing responsibilities doesn't make us carefree because like it or not the work we escaped will be there waiting for us unless it's been replaced by a pink slip. We don't think our metaphors will be among those trampled on the now famous cutting room floor. We say this because we are not creating these metaphors for literary effect. We use them to help you get to where you want to be. We offer them as guides for you to consider and hopefully use.

We have chosen a number of famous freeway events. We will tell you about the event. We will share Jeff's experiences as he reported the event. We will then present a life situation related metaphorically to the freeway event. Sometimes our biggest traffic jams are the ones we encounter in our daily lives. We'll help you either avoid those or get out of them so you can ultimately be where you want to be in your life as well as on the road.

4

FREEWAY HELPERS AND LIFE LESSONS

AVIGATING OUR LIVES IS a lot like driving on the Los Angeles Freeway system. If we stick with the metaphor that freeway experiences equal or greatly resemble life experiences we quickly discover that Los Angeles freeways have some very helpful things going on. We can learn from them and then we can figure out how to apply them to our daily lives so that, yes, we can really get to where we want to be.

Botts Dots

Imagine a warning system to tell us when we're straying off our chosen path. Imagine going a little off track and we hear and feel the warning sound and the vibration of wheels hitting little raised, round, non-reflective, raised pavement marker dots. We don't have those to keep us headed in the right direction in our lives but we do have them on our freeways. Botts dots, they're called. They are named after Dr. Elbert Dysart Botts, an engineer for the California Department of Transportation (Caltrans). Botts supervised a Caltrans research project charged with finding a way to increase the paint life of the road striping. Little did he know that his little dots would save lives by alerting the driver who wandered a little out of the lane when sleepy or distracted!

Those dots are used throughout this country and even in some foreign countries. What Dr. Botts didn't invent was a warning device for our inner journeys or our off the road life journeys. We have to create our own rumble strips. We can do it. It would be so nice to have some sort of built in, automatic warning that we're going off track.

We can build upon the warnings created by Dr. Botts. For example, you might also consider creating a self-check list. Before Jeff and his pilot take off, the pilot goes through an inspection checklist to make sure the plane is safe to fly and Jeff checks his scanners and radios to make sure he's ready to report. We believe that all of us would benefit from a similar daily checklist.

Let's give it a try right now. Write down a few things that you need to do every day to keep you on the right path for your well-being. You might put down things like exercise, listen to music, meditate, brush the dog, study for that test, write in a journal, take a bubble bath—whatever you need to do to keep yourself intact. I maintain such a list. I revisit it regularly just to make sure I'm tending to my own needs. Go ahead. Make your list. There's no right or wrong on your "Personal Botts Dots List" as long as the items on your list aren't harmful to you or to any other living being.

Check your list regularly. If you aren't doing the things on your list then you aren't tending to yourself. You aren't doing what you need to do for yourself. When you get used to this type of self- care you will begin to feel the ride getting rough and hear the sounds of you running over those Botts Dots as you drift off course.

Your self-care list can help you stay on the path you want to travel. Use it.

Freeway Service Patrol

The Freeway Service Patrol (FSP) was one of THE best things to happen to Los Angeles Freeways. FSP was a parting gift from Tom Bradley just before he stepped down as mayor of Los Angeles. Before its creation, freeway problems that re-quired tow trucks were done mostly by private garages with a response time of approximately FOREVER!

The FSP is a joint program provided by the California De-partment of Transportation (Caltrans), the California High-way Patrol (CHP) and the local transportation agency. It's a free service of privately owned tow trucks that patrol desig-nated routes on congested California freeways. Its goal is to help drivers get to where they want to go by keeping traffic moving and drivers safe. Each year the FSP assists about 650,000 drivers. There are limits to what FSP can do. But the point is that it helps us get to where we want to go. It's kind of like having a best friend in the lane next to us just in case we need some help. In our lives off of the freeways we still need some sort of FSP. Since we don't have personal FSP programs we can create something similar. We can develop a system of buddies. As much as we might wish to be self-re-liant we really aren't. We are social creatures living in social situations. We need each other. As long as that's the way things are, we suggest creating and maintaining good, strong, reliable social support systems—friends, family members, or colleagues at work.

Ask those people you trust to let you know if they notice that you are going off path. Since you trust them and you've asked them to do this for you, believe them if they tell you that you are seeming to be easily angered or not interested in things that previously thrilled you. Once you've let that important feedback seep into your consciousness, problem solve with them ways to get back on track.

That system would be called our Social Support System— Our S-Cubed or our Triple S or whatever we want to call it. The purpose of this system wouldn't be to bring us a gallon of gas when we've run out on The 210. In California that's what the FSP does so we don't need to duplicate a good thing. The purpose of our SSS might be to come on over when we need to talk. Or maybe to tell us we're doing a good job. Or maybe just to sit with us when we're feeling down. Another name for that Social Support System might be simply friends or family. Use them. And a heads up here. Be there for them, too.

Just for fun, write down the names of three people you might consider asking to be part of your SSS. We think it's important to write things down so we can remember or consider some other time.

1. ....

2. ....

3. ....

Now you have a start on your SSS. Sometimes you don't need a whole posse. Just a couple of people can make a world of difference.

SigAlerts

By 1950 Los Angeles traffic was already famous for accidents and traffic jams. The Los Angeles Police Department's phone lines were continually swamped by calls from radio stations asking for traffic updates. The LAPD Officers throughout the days and nights kept repeating the same information over and over. Clearly the system wasn't working.

Enter Loyd C. "Sig" Sigmon. During World War II "Sig" served in the United States Army Signal Corps on the staff of General Dwight D. Eisenhower. By the time the LAPD phone lines were swamped with calls for traffic information, Sig was the executive vice president of Golden West Broadcasters' Los Angeles Radio Station KMPC. He doubtless wasn't too thrilled with all the phone line tie ups either and decided to fix the situation once and for all. He developed a system which, in the most simplified explanation possible, allowed LAPD to notify area radio stations of heavy traffic situations. The current California Highway Patrol definition of a SigAlert is "any unplanned event that causes the closing of one lane of traffic for 30 minutes or more". Then LAPD Chief William H. Parker, skeptical of the new system's efficacy, gave it the name SigAlert possibly to distance himself from it as much as possible.

Today versions of the SigAlert are used throughout the country. Wouldn't it be great if we had such a system to warn us that we are putting too much on our plates and risk feeling overwhelmed by life? We don't have one but we can create our own. It's up to us to recognize our warning signs. We can all learn to do just that. Stick with us.

Traffic Breaks

One of the most amazing things that can happen on a Los Angeles freeway is the traffic break. A traffic break can be requested by the Freeway Service Patrol or can be initiated by the California Highway Patrol. If it starts with the FSP (Freeway Service Patrol) then the request goes to the California Highway Patrol. Either way, the traffic break is done by the CHP. The purpose of the traffic break is to bring freeway traffic to a stop so that the FSP or the CHP can remove debris from the roadway, tow a vehicle to the shoulder or off the freeway, get to a vehicle, or any other activity that requires a person out of the vehicle and onto the asphalt. At times depending on CHP manpower the traffic break can take a while but here's what a traffic break looks like. The officer drives onto the freeway in question and when close to the 'incident' or the 'debris' or the 'whatever' (about 1/2 mile away) starts driving back and forth across all lanes of traffic with the cruisers emergency lights on to slow, then stop all traffic. Sometimes the savvy FSP driver will see this coming from behind, go into lanes and start the process of clearing whatever the problem is. Usually this whole procedure takes just minutes. The problem is removed and all lanes open again. It's a fascinating display of expertise and patience.

Jeff frequently jokes with members of the CHP at meetings or other events about how they keep their weapons holstered when a lot of drivers will not heed to their wishes to stop. He often watches this from the air. The process starts and finally the officer is now stopped.

All lights are flashing, the cruiser is sideways on the freeway and the officer exits the vehicle to assist the driver in need or help the FSP driver when inevitably someone goes blasting through putting everyone in harm's way only to finally say to the officer when stopped (sometimes after a short chase), "Oh you wanted ME to stop too?"

At meetings they all laugh but it's quite scary to watch from the air and is really serious for the officers when it happens. And it happens every day. Traffic breaks are for everyone and, yes, everyone is expected to stop.

Traffic breaks are wonderful. Everything comes, eventually, to a complete stop. They present an opportunity to pause, remove the hazards, and begin again. That's a glory of the Los Angeles freeway system. The problem is, though, that in our lives we don't have the FSP or the CHP to force us to slow down or to come to a complete stop, regroup and hit the road again. We have to learn to recognize the hazards, to come to the stop, to clear the obstacles, and to start again. We can learn to do that, though.

You've already started the learning process with Botts Dots and the Freeway Service Patrol and the SigAlert. It's not easy to slow down or come to a complete stop. We know that. Sometimes, though, it is absolutely necessary if we are going to correct our current course and get back on our path.

Stick with us and we'll help you.

Detours

Detours can be a nuisance. There we are on our way to wherever we want to go and all of a sudden we have to turn back or take another route. As inconvenient as they may be, detours help keep us safe. The road is closed for a reason. Even understanding the purpose of the detour, change is seldom easy.

Often on the road the detour signs clearly guide us around the hazard and put us back on a safer route. We generally drive on to our intended destination. Off the road and in life we lack such clear warnings to change routes and rarely are we given signs along the way to help guide us along the new path. All too often when we must change plans we wind up somewhere unexpected. We wind up where we didn't want to go.

There are no laws reminding us to change life goals or take a different route to the original goals. We need to create those self-regulating mechanisms ourselves. Changing directions or destinations is really hard.

For many novice airplane pilots the most difficult in the air maneuver to learn is the 180-degree turn. Inexperienced pilots, despite every imaginable warning signal, will maintain straight ahead direction until the bitter end. Often, sadly, the bitter end is a fatal crash.

Traveling on the road and in life demands attention. While we don't have cockpit or dashboard warning lights and bells, we do have our instincts. Pilots, despite the numbers of instruments they may have in the cockpit, fly by the seat of their pants. They feel the airplane's position and speed. They are not passengers. They are the pilots. Their job is to fly the plane. In order to do that they must feel the plane. We fly our life planes. We drive our life vehicles. Our challenge is to do so using our minds, our emotions, and the seats of our pants.

How do we know when to change? We keep in constant touch with our thoughts and our emotions. We develop an awareness of the hair on our arms and on the back of our necks. We listen to our guts. We live by the seat of our pants.

In the pages that follow we will help you develop that awareness and that ability. Change is hard. Taking alternate routes and developing new goals is also difficult. By planning for both possibilities we can avoid spinning out of control.

Stick with us and we'll help you gain better control and maintain forward progress. Instead of zig zagging along you'll be able to choose a straight line to get where you want to be.

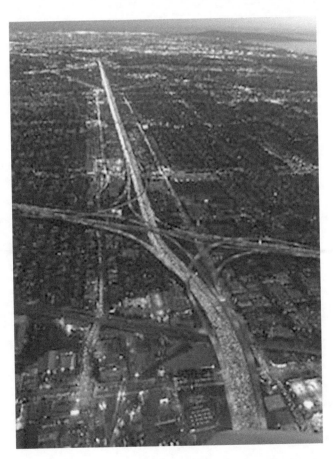

5.

KNOW WHERE YOU WANT TO GO AND HOW TO GET THERE

WHEN WAS THE LAST time you tried to buy a road map? Not too long ago we could go to any gas station or auto club or drug store or grocery store and easily choose a road map from a large selection. These days buying a map isn't so easy. If we want to locate a good café in Paris we can select from several maps of downtown Paris in just about any bookstore. However, trying to locate a passable route from Baltimore to Boston with a road map is becoming just about impossible.

Global Positioning Systems (GPSs) are pervasive and the majority of travelers rely on them. They come with our cell phones. They are already on the dashboards of our newer vehicles or a portable one can be mounted on the dashboard of any vehicle. They are in many ways miracles of navigation. Why, we don't even have to think about where we are going in order to arrive at our destination. And that is why we worry about exclusive use of any type of GPS. Research indicates that when used as our only navigational mechanism, the Global Positioning System changes the very structure of our brains.

How many times has this happened to you? You're driving along not paying much attention to the road and all of a sudden you realize that you've been on autopilot for the past several miles. You have no idea how you got to where you are at that moment. It's pretty scary, isn't it? Indications are that when we rely on our GPS we are generally on autopilot. Our brains aren't doing much of the navigating.

We drive along in a pseudo brain-dead state not paying attention to our surroundings. We have placed all of our trust in the wisdom of our GPS. Often that trust leads us to misadventures and even to tragedies. A New Jersey businessman visiting Iceland tried driving from the airport to a nearby hotel guided only by the information he put into his GPS. Many hours and 250 miles later he stopped at a fishing village in the Arctic Circle to ask for directions. A Japanese tourist in Australia drove into the Pacific Ocean because his GPS told him he was on a road instead of a beach. A man in West Yorkshire, England, kept following the path that his GPS insisted was a road until he nearly drove off a cliff. People drive down stairways, off bridges, and follow roads no longer in use to their deaths because they have placed their complete faith in the accuracy of their GPS and ignored the detour signs or the road closure signs.

Jeff and Mary love maps. They also love Global Positioning Systems. They believe, though, that it is important to not toss one in the trash for love of the other. When we use a map we force our brains to work—to pay attention.

Shortly after graduating from Arizona State University with a Bachelor's Degree in Secondary Education, Mary taught sixth grade geography in a small Arizona town. Never a strict adherent to the syllabus, she decided that more important than memorizing the average annual rainfall in Nairobi, Kenya, was the ability to read a road map. She also believed that her students should learn to draw their own maps. Just for fun, pretend that you are in that sixth grade geography class. Your assignment is to draw a map. Choose someplace in your city with which you are familiar. Let's say the store where you shop for groceries or where you go for coffee or breakfast. Draw a map showing a route from your home to that store or restaurant. It doesn't have to be to scale and it doesn't have to be pretty. Just give it a try.

Good work. Now take another look at your map. If you followed your route would you get home? Great. You did well. Now take another look at it. Try to remember any landmarks or visual clues along the way. Indicate those on your map, too. Is there a flagpole somewhere between your house and the store? What about an interesting building? Without the step-by-step directions provided by the GPS, we travel from place to place using landmarks and visual clues. Our brains create their own cognitive maps.

You've all heard stories of the traveling salesman who out in the country loses his way. He stops to ask a farmer for directions to the small hotel down the road in the next town. The farmer's response goes something like this:

"Well, you see that old mailbox down the road? Go past it and then turn left close to the broken gate. Keep going on past the yellow barn and then when you see the flagpole in Belle Bakers's yard get ready to turn right. Keep on that road until you go past the Post Office. Your hotel is just down the road."

In order to follow those directions and get to his hotel, the salesman had to observe and think. He had to pay attention to his surroundings and look for (1) that old mailbox (2) the broken gate (3) the yellow barn (4) the flagpole and (5) the Post Office. The hippocampus in the temporal lobe of the traveling salesman's brain got a good workout following those directions. The salesman was forced to 'learn' how to get to his hotel and in that learning process engaged in the cognitive process of mental mapping.

The hippocampus is involved in memory and in navigation processes. It helps us find new routes and identify short cuts. Researchers at Canada's McGill University suggest that exclusive dependence on GPS for navigation may have a negative effect on brain function by decreasing the amount of grey matter in the hippocampus. The hippocampus is one of the first parts of the brain to be affected by Alzheimer's disease, which impairs not only memory but also spatial orientation. Just as we want to take good care of our hearts, we want to take good care of our brains. We can do that by engaging in activities that challenge us to remember and think and problem solve.

McGill University neuroscientist Veronique Bohbot suggests that people who just follow directions without thought or question have less gray matter in their hippocampus. This suggests that we use our GPS to get us to a new destination but then shut it off on the return trip thus forcing our brains to use mental mapping and spatial memory.

In 1948 University of California at Berkeley psychologist Edward Tolman studied the behavior of rats in mazes to determine that rats could develop cognitive 'strip maps' that limited spatial relationships between only two points. The rats could also develop much broader cognitive maps showing the spatial relationships of the entire maze. Studies at the University of Freiburg's Center for Cognitive Science indicate that exclusive GPS use impairs our ability to create mental maps of the 'big picture' and reduces us to a strip-map worldview both literal and metaphorical. Confined to the strip map worldview, unable to see the bigger picture, we are more likely to ignore the detour sign and drive off the cliff. Seeing the bigger picture is important not only on the road but also in all of life. With only a strip-map understanding, we are more likely to judge our neighbors harshly while ignoring the bigger maze in which we all try to find our way.

Further informing the self-centric, strip map worldview is the reality that our GPS constantly reorients itself to put us in the center of the universe. We never have to figure out where we are because we are right there in the middle of everything. As much as this information may wound, we aren't really the center of the universe. You may not want to hear this, either, but it's really important for us to keep figuring out how to get to where we want to be on our own. Yes, we will make mistakes. We will take wrong turns on the road and in life. However, by remembering the routes that took us to where we didn't want to be we can avoid similar paths in the future. That can't happen, though, unless we remember the landmarks and the visual clues along the way.

Jeff often talks about the value of keeping a map folded up in our windshield visor. Even with a GPS, that map can be a lifesaver. And we know that using only our GPS can impair our ability to think and chart alternate routes. So let's hang on to both of our navigational tools while always remembering that the most important tool we have is our brains. Let's use them wisely.

We've talked a lot about navigation. However, before we can navigate anyplace we must figure out where we want to go. That's really the hard part. While we get it that starting a road trip with no destination in mind would be at best frivolous, how many of us make plans for our life destinations? Do you really have a plan for the next year? Or for the next five years? We can't go to an auto club and get a TripTik for our lives. We have to figure that out on our own. Right now are you living the life you want to live? Are you doing the work of your dreams? Trust us. It is never too late to change routes or to chart new routes. Regardless of your age or your expertise you can start moving toward where you want your life to be.

Take a minute now to jot down some things you like to do or some things you'd like to become.

....

....

....

....

Now just like the map you drew from the grocery store to your home, you can draw a map charting the route to accomplishing or obtaining some of those things on your list. Don't forget to break down the route into very small, achievable steps. This is just like driving from New York City to Philadelphia. We don't say we're going to get in the car and arrive in Philadelphia. We need to plan our route and know that there will be pit stops and traffic and maybe even an occasional delay. We also know that we will arrive eventually.

So go ahead. Choose one thing from the list you made and see if you can break it down to as many achievable tasks as possible.

....

....

....

....

Off you go, now. Don't forget to pack snacks and take time to enjoy the scenery.

6

THE MAJOR FREEWAY EVENTS AND WHAT WE CAN LEARN FROM THEM

FOR THE PURPOSES OF description and learning, we've chosen ten major freeway events to share with you. Some occurred on an actual freeway. Other events significantly impacted freeway traffic even though they did not take place on any Los Angeles area freeway. All of these ten events classified as 'Breaking News' and Jeff reported on each one. Mary was impacted either directly or indirectly by each of these events as were thousands upon thousands of other Southern California residents and visitors.

We share these events with you to provide a glimpse into the amazing history of the Los Angeles freeway, to illustrate the place automobile travel holds in our lives, and to give you tools for not only safer travel but also more satisfying and happier living. We learn as we go. Our hope is that these pages will help your learning.

. . .

CRANE COLLAPSE IN THE CAHUENGA PASS

One March day in 1998 on the Hollywood Freeway in the Cahuenga Pass, the driver of a construction vehicle lost control in the southbound lanes. The vehicle jack-knifed and a crane being towed by the vehicle toppled over. This accident resulted in one of the worst traffic jams in the infamous Los Angeles freeway history.

The crane came to rest lying across all northbound lanes and most of the southbound lanes. An extraordinary number of first responders arrived almost immediately. The driver of one vehicle was pronounced dead at the scene. Paramedics tended to many more injured. A medical triage became quickly operational and a massive variety of emergency equipment arrived almost before the dust had settled. The California Highway patrol and other jurisdictions arrived on the scene in what seemed like an endless stream of first responders.

The Hollywood Freeway (The 101) connects downtown Los Angeles and the San Fernando Valley. You may recall that the Arroyo Seco Parkway is the oldest and the Hollywood Freeway is the second oldest in the Southern California freeway system. You've also probably seen the downtown Los Angeles part of this freeway in a lot of pictures of the famous Four Level Interchange used to illustrate the Los Angeles lure of automobiles in motion.

This accident took place in a section of that freeway steeped in history and legend. The Cahuenga Pass (pronounced Ka-wane-ga) was the site of two major battles. The first was the Battle of Cahuenga Pass in 1831 between local settlers and the army of the Mexican appointed governor. Two people died in that fight. The second was the Battle of Providencia in 1845 between locals over whether to secede from Mexico. A horse and a mule died in that fight. Once in a while even today a cannon ball is found during construction excavations to remind us that serious stuff happened in that pass. The old El Camino Real went through that pass. It's also rumored that a treasure of gold is buried somewhere in the pass.

The Hollywood Freeway goes through this famous Cahuenga Pass where it is four lanes going in each direction. And it's in a canyon so things feel pretty close together. This is the place where the construction crane collapsed and eventually blocked all eight lanes of the Hollywood Freeway. Remember that this freeway is a lifeline between the Valley and downtown Los Angeles.

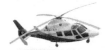 **IN THE AIR WITH JEFF!**

"Okay, listen up! This is a major event, unfolding right now!" I've been told by radio veterans—especially program directors—that those words get attention. When people hear me say them on the radio they really listen. Unfortunately I've had to use that opening in far too many traffic reports.

On this particular day, though, people either in the Cahuenga Pass or about to enter it knew when they heard my words that change was about to happen. When I spoke those words I knew that this crash was about to affect thousands of commuters.

The Cahuenga Pass became inaccessible in both directions. News of the accident and its resulting traffic jam was immediately broadcast on all area television and radio stations. News helicopters hovered overhead broadcasting last minute developments. Despite the immediate and ubiquitous news flashes, the traffic jam grew until it eventually stretched several miles in both directions. For hours commuters sat in their cars or on the hoods of their cars waiting as more and more drivers, despite the constant warnings to stay away from the Hollywood Freeway, inched down on ramps to join the quagmire of cars. All this while many area surface streets remained relatively uncongested. One might reasonably ask why people chose to get onto a freeway and sit immobilized in traffic for hours instead of taking alternate routes, especially since the news media was not only urging people to do so but was, in fact, educating them on how to get to those alternate routes. Responses to the question of "Why did you choose to get on an unusable freeway and sit for hours going nowhere?" might have included, "Because this is the way I always go home." or "I didn't know what the other routes were like." or "I wasn't sure those other routes would be any better." And so they sat motionless for hours playing their roles of quintessentially perfect commuters as though they had no voice or choice in the matter.

That afternoon lives in my mind as the SigAlert that came closest to bringing traffic to a halt and a city to its knees. This was a wreck that sprawled and bottled up everything in that pass. For hours few cars moved. Surface streets were gridlocked. Surrounding freeways were backed up. And some children weren't picked up from school until late evening.

In broad daylight all I saw at first was an almost blinding sea of flashing, red emergency lights. This is all horrendous enough for those directly involved but what was unfolding rapidly for drivers headed from all points of the compass, particularly drivers headed North through the Cahuenga Pass just before the afternoon commute, was absolute chaos. A major freeway was closed. This wasn't a ladder in a lane or a stalled car. This wasn't a fender bender or a jack-knifed big rig in all three lanes in the same direction of a freeway. This was an entire freeway closed in both directions. One side of a Los Angeles freeway closed during rush hour can back traffic up for ten miles in a matter of just twenty minutes.

The moment I absorbed the scene below me I knew that I could help. My number one task from that moment on was to start drivers thinking about and taking alternative routes. Everyone in the Los Angeles basin needed to stop thinking 'freeway' because this accident quickly impacted the entire city. The Hollywood Freeway was closed.

From the moment I first started flying above the traffic and reporting on it, I have been astonished by the overwhelming percentage of drivers who keep getting on a freeway that is clearly stopped. And as soon as they get on they, too, stop. Even when on-ramps are visibly backed up onto the surface streets many drivers still struggle to get on the closed freeway only to sit in their cars.

For a considerable length of time after this particular accident there were a lot of alternate routes available. For a whole lot of reasons, though, people just weren't taking them. Instead, drivers just kept heading for the Cahuenga Pass even though there was clearly no way to get through it.

Sometimes even in this time of a GPS on every electronic device the most valuable tool to have with you is a map tucked up behind your visor. We seem to use the same freeways and surface streets day in and day out almost like their use is mandatory.

Plans B, C and D are essential not just conceptually but

actually. We have to know other ways to get to where we want to go. With a little help you can take a path you never took before and be so pleasantly surprised and proud of yourself for pulling it all off. It's okay not to use the freeway!!!!

Here's something else to consider. Sometimes just pulling off the road and having a long cup of coffee or dinner will help you through the bedlam. Unless you've got some pressing reason to be at your destination at a specific time give yourself and the traffic a break. Get off the freeway or the grid locked street and give yourself a time out. Trust me. You won't regret it. Make the call so the folks at home or at work won't worry too much and enjoy the coffee.

A few months after this crane event played out, the radio station I was working for forwarded an envelope to me. Inside was a small thank you note in which a woman described using a rather obscure but direct alternate route I was looking at and describing. At the time I was urging people to take it, the route was relatively empty going over the Hollywood Hills and into the San Fernando Valley. The woman forced herself to get out of her comfort zone and give it a try. It worked as advertised and most important got the woman to her anxious and worried child still waiting at school. Nice!!! There are ways around freeway problems in Los Angeles. All you have to do is learn them and do something proactive and take a different path!

 ## ON THE GROUND WITH MARY!

Our first learning opportunity involves change. We're beginning with change because this book is all about change. We are suggesting that if you aren't getting to where you want to be you might consider making some changes in the way you are doing what you do. If I'm going around in circles and I want to actually get someplace, then I'm going to have to either change my route or decide that going around in circles is what I wanted after all. So we start with change.

The crane collapse was a terrible accident that killed and injured. It also tied up traffic for hours and almost stopped a city. The traffic tie-ups right after the accident were unavoidable. People were in the pass and they were stopped. However, after the news of the accident got out much of the gridlock could have been avoided. Jeff wasn't the only reporter in the sky asking, begging, and demanding people to take an alternate route. There were plenty of other folks up there doing pretty much the same thing. He was just doing it better than all of the other reporters.

Drivers didn't keep heading into the Pass to spite Jeff or to deliberately make matters worse. They did it because that was their route. That was the way they went to work or ran the errands or came home from work or made the deliveries. Every day that was the route they took.

Maybe they didn't know any alternate routes. Maybe they weren't listening to their radios. Surely at some point, though, even miles from the accident they could see that traffic was at an all time slow crawl. That would have been a good time to turn on the radio or take a different path. For the most part, though, and for most of that day folks just kept heading on into the Cahuenga Pass. So if they weren't out to get Jeff and if they weren't deliberately trying to make things worse, what was going on?

Change is really hard. The longer we repeat the same activity or the same routine or the same route the harder making a change becomes. It's almost like we create our own ruts and can't figure out how to climb out of them.

The Oregon Trail is a perfect example of such ruts. It stretched over two thousand miles to connect the Missouri River to the valleys of what would become the state of Oregon. Created by fur trappers in the early 1800s, it was originally passable only on foot or horseback. As westward migration became a fact of life, the trail was cleared until it was wide enough for wagons. You've seen depictions of those wagons in hundreds of movies. They were the covered, Conestoga wagons with their big wheels and insides packed with everything a family could conceivably need in its new home. Oxen, mules or maybe on occasion horses pulled those wagons. On a good day, the wagons averaged a speed of about two miles an hour.

Within twenty years about 400,000 wagons traveled west on the Oregon Trail. That's a lot of wheels and hooves. By 1869 railroads practically put the Oregon Trail out of business. These days we call that same route Interstate 80 and in places it runs pretty close to the original trail.

Even though at no time could the wagon trip on the Oregon Trail be called easy or comfortable, those first few wagons had a really rough time of it because, well, they were the first. The westward bound settlers had to break in the trail, so to speak. After a few thousand wagons, though, the trail was pretty much broken in and, in fact, was becoming rutted.

Today there's a park about five miles south of Guernsey, Wyoming, along the North Platte River. In 1966 that park was designated a National Historic Landmark and its sole purpose is to preserve the ruts created by the wagons and the animals and the people going west on the Oregon Trail. Some of those ruts are six feet deep.

Think back to those first wagons. They were the first. There weren't any ruts. There was perhaps a cleared space. Some of the big boulders were moved to the side but those first wagons could even veer off the trail a bit if the animals or the people wanted to do such a thing. It might not have been safe but it could be done. There was choice. There was freedom. Now think of those last hundred thousand or so wagons. In places they were moving along in ruts sometimes six feet deep.

What were the chances of changing directions for those folks? Change was not very likely. Once those wagons were in a six-foot deep rut they were pretty much stuck there. Such a situation might feel pretty safe. No decisions were needed because once the wagon was in the rut there was no getting out until the rut ended. Sometimes not having to decide can seem like an okay place to be. On the other hand, not being able to make a change can also be risky. What if there was trouble ahead and there you were in your Conestoga wagon stuck in a six-foot deep rut. They kept going that way because that was their route. That was the way they went to get to Oregon.

Those Oregon Trail ruts were made by hundreds of thousands of hooves and feet and wagons and not just by one wagon filled with one family pulled by one team. In all likelihood the ruts would have gotten just as deep if only one wagon had gone back and forth endlessly for twenty or so years and not just because even one of those wagons weighed five or six tons when full but because that's what happens when we endlessly repeat the same thing over and over again.

Change is hard anyway but when we're stuck in ruts of our own making it can seem practically impossible. Consider the

Cahuenga Pass and all of those drivers who just kept trying to get through only to sit motionless for hours. Why were they doing that? Because that was their route and they couldn't get out of their daily ruts.

Come to find out our brains are a lot like the Oregon Trail. Think of the dirt or mud or sand of that trail. It was the repetition of those heavy wagons and those hooves and those people going over and over the same dirt that made the ruts. Our brains are made of matter a lot softer than the ground of the Oregon Trail. A part of our brain is called our neural pathways.

Neural pathways are like interstate highways (Interstate 80 for example) of nerve cells. Instead of moving wagons full of the requirements for new lives on the Oregon Trail or trucks full of food or televisions on I-80, our neural pathways move messages.

"Foot to brain. Some idiot is standing on me and I'm hurting. Pain. Pain. Pain."

"Hands on steering wheel to brain. I'm turning left because that's the way I always turn and I feel safer doing what I always do."

But I've oversimplified. Clearly the messages transmitted via our neural pathways are considerably more complicated and probably not transmitted in words or sentences. However, my point is that we can slow down or stop the effectiveness of those pathways with repetition.

We always turn left because that's the route we take to wherever. Over and over again until the pathways become increasingly solid and increasingly rutted until one day you hear Jeff begging you to take an alternate route and you simply can't make the change. Or until one day you can't help but notice that the traffic hasn't moved for quite some time and even though you see an opportunity to go another way you just can't quite climb that six-foot deep rut and change.

And as it works out repetition whether it be thought or behavior can make ruts in those neural pathways. The longer we repeat that same thought or behavior the deeper those ruts become until ultimately we have a really tough time climbing out of them.

Unlike those six-foot deep ruts on the Oregon Trail, though, our brains have a thing called neuroplasticity. We can get out of those mind ruts or at least get them under control. When we train our brains to think different thoughts and engage in different behaviors it's almost like we are re-wiring them. Brain re-wiring doesn't require an electrician's license or any type of special training. It does, though, require some determination, a little planning and maybe some creativity.

Research indicates that one first step for safe and effective brain re-wiring is to start doing everyday things differently. Here are some examples: If you ordinarily brush your teeth with your right hand start using your left hand or the other way around. Try walking across a room backwards. And horror of horrors, try taking a different route to work or the grocery store or the gym. You might even try eating dessert first. I'm not sure doing so will un-rut your brain but it might be fun anyway. Also, if you find out you don't like liver and onions after all you will at least have had dessert.

Doing these everyday things differently probably won't create significant changes in your life. It will, however, start removing those ruts from that neural transmitter super highway. While you're walking backwards across your living room, take a second to consider those New Years' resolutions you make every December 31st. Have you ever kept them long enough to even begin working out more often? How many times did you go to the gym before tossing in the towel? Yeah, me too. I've got nothing against gym memberships but I think the gyms make most of their money from people who join in late December or early January, go a few times, and then never go back. Somewhere there is a huge stack of towels from all those of us who have tossed it in.

Write down a couple of resolutions for change that you made either recently or quite a while back. Go on. We're not looking. We're certainly not judging, either. We have lists of things we meant to change or start or finish so long you wouldn't believe we even thought of that stuff. In fact I'll write down a couple of my annual resolutions just to help you feel less silly and also to remind you that we all go through this.

1. Lose weight. 2. Write more. 3. Do more serious reading.

....

....

....

....

How did your plans for change work out? I can tell you that mine didn't work out and now I know why. They were not clearly defined. They tried to accomplish too much and/or they are generally completely unrealistic.

Take another look at the resolutions I made that year and every year for a lot of years. At first glance they seem like perfectly fine resolutions that focus on improving body and mind and career. So what happened? First of all, they are really vague. How much weight do I want to lose? How much more do I want to write? And what on earth is my definition of serious reading? Also, how much is more? See? I wouldn't even know if or when I had met those goals but instead of calling myself a success after one pound lost or one word written or one page read, I'm going to call myself a colossal failure because I didn't lose or write or read enough even though I never said how much would be enough to begin with!

Okay, so if you want to make changes try to be as specific as possible. For example, let's take my second resolution. What would have happened if I had written it like this? "For the next thirty days I will write a minimum of three pages per day on any project." That's pretty specific. And I could actually probably achieve that goal and finally be able to scratch that resolution off the endlessly repeating list of resolutions.

Change is hard because we make our own six-foot deep ruts and also because once we decide to make some sort of change we have trouble figuring out how go about making that change. Also sometimes we aren't even sure we want to change anything.

A lot of people have spent a lot of time studying change and they have created different models to illustrate the stages of change. All of those models boil down to pretty much the same stages.

1. We're not even thinking about change.
2. We're beginning to think about change but we're still undecided.
3. We might make some changes but right now we're just testing the waters.
4. We've made the change and we're practicing the new behavior.
5. We're trying to keep the change we made.

Most of those change models also make room for slipping back to doing what we were doing before we made the change. That happens and hopefully when it does we can get back on track and continue with the change. Take a look at those stages of change again. We're not going to make changes in our lives until we're ready and that happens somewhere between stages three and stage four.

If we're stuck in our brain ruts it could take a really long time to move on to stage four. And sometimes we don't have that much time. For example, when Jeff says, "Listen up! This is a major event. Don't go into the Cahuenga Pass," we need to make some quick decisions. We need to race through stages one, two and three and get off the 101 freeway to take another route. So let's practice some more. Think of some changes you are considering and try to figure out where are you in the process. It's important to know where we are so we can move ahead. Go ahead. Take some time right now and list two or three changes you're thinking about. Just to clarify, you are only thinking about making these changes. You haven't got a plan. You've only got thoughts.

1. ....

2. ....

3. ....

The next challenge is probably simpler than listing the things you might like to change. Now, please list reasons for not making the change or changes. Some of the reasons might be that the change is too complicated, that it won't work, that it costs too much, that people will laugh, or it's too much to take on. Take a minute, though, and find your own reasons for not changing.

My reasons for not making any changes are:

....

....

....

....

....

....

....

....

Be honest. Isn't it easier to list reasons for not making any changes? It's always so much easier for me to not make a change in my behavior or my routines. And then I'm off the hook. I don't have to go any further. Game over. I don't even have to worry about failing because I'm not going to try.

However, if I remember those stages of change I might also remember that during the contemplation stage I'm ambivalent. I'm sitting on the fence. It's easy to fall off the fence and land on the side of not making any change. All it takes is a little shove from the list you made above.

So in addition to understanding that there are stages of change, it's also useful to understand that there are obstacles to change. Knowing the obstacles helps us overcome them or at least work around them.

Let's make one more list. Think again of the changes you might begin to think about making. Got it? Okay. Now jot a few reasons for changing.

My reasons for changing are:

....

....

....

....

....

....

....

....

Now compare your two lists. If there are more reasons for not making any change or if the reasons for not making any change are more compelling, then mission accomplished. It's not time to make the change or there's no reason to make it. On the other hand, if the reasons for making the change outnumber the reasons for not making it or if they are more compelling, then mission also accomplished. It's time to make a change.

Once you've decided to make that change it's important to understand a couple of other things. The way things were is a really powerful force. The way things were might also be called the status quo or the steady state. Regardless of how much we want change, we don't like it when it's happening. Change, well, changes everything. That's why it's so hard for organizations or cultures or countries to implement change. With change comes a certain amount of chaos. We aren't what we were and we don't know who we will become.

Let's take my resolution to lose weight. I've made the decision and I've even broken the goal down into baby steps—manageable smaller goals that I know I can achieve. I'm well on my way to losing weight. The trouble is, though, that this is new territory for me. I'm exercising and I'm changing the way I eat and that's kind of scary.

My discomfort and uncertainty make it easier—more comfortable, more certain—to stop the changes that were leading me to that uncertain albeit healthier new me. And so I stop exercising and forget all about that new way of eating. Now I'm me again and I'm comfortable except that, once again, I've failed to meet my goal.

All living systems including you and I want to maintain that steady state—that status quo. Intellectually we understand that without change there can be no progress. So the changes we choose might be easier if we accept that with change comes inevitable but temporary instability. We will regain our balance and a new steady state if we just keep choosing the changes we chose to begin with. If I keep eating a healthy breakfast I will eventually be more uncomfortable with my breakfast doughnut than I was during that unstable time of change. When that happens I will know that I have created a new status quo—a new steady state.

There are a couple of other things that might make change difficult. Knowing the obstacles can help us overcome them or at least work around them. So in addition to the power of the status quo trying to pull you backwards to the way things were, fear can slow your change down—fear of change, fear of the unknown, just fear. And the more we understand about fear the more likely we are to manage it and move through it. Another obstacle to change is the feelings we experience when we start thinking about or implementing the changes we have chosen to make. We also have thoughts about change and those thoughts will influence what we are feeling about the change. For example, if I think that I will fail I am going to feel anxious or sad. I might not even try to make changes. On the other hand, if I think that I will succeed and enjoy my weight loss journey, for example, I will have feelings based on those thoughts, which might include optimism and confidence. Bottom line is that if we are careful choosing our thoughts about change, we are more likely to keep the changes we have chosen.

Here's another aspect of change worthy of consideration. Some things we can change and some things we cannot change. It's really important to know which is which. We can change our thoughts and our behaviors. We can change our habits and, yes, we can even change the way we feel about change. We can change some things we at one time believed impossible. There are, though, limitations on what we can change. I can't, for example, change my age. I was born on a specific date. However, I can change the way I age and the way I feel about aging. And here's another amazing thing about change. One change changes everything. When I start eating healthy foods and exercising and losing weight I'll discover that more has changed in my life than breakfast. My self-confidence, my self-esteem, my energy level, my physical and mental health may all change for the better.

Now we know that if we keep doing the same things over and over we run the risk of making ruts in our brain pretty much like those ruts on the Oregon Trail. We also know that we can soften up and get rid of those brain ruts by changing our daily routines. We also know that we can make significant changes in our lives by mapping out the routes to those changes. We are all in charge of the changes we choose to make.

RIOTS AFTER THE RODNEY KING VERDICT

On March 3, 1991, Rodney King led police on a high speed chase through Los Angeles County. When the chase eventually ended, King resisted arrest. He was beaten by Los Angeles police officers. The event was filmed with a personal video camera. The public release of the video caused outrage on a national level as well as a debate on police brutality. Rodney King, who was taken into custody the night of the beating, was released without charges. On March 15th Sergeant Stacey Koon and Officers Laurence Powell, Theodore Briseno and Timothy Wind were indicted by a grand jury and each charged with assault with a deadly weapon and excessive use of force. Powell and Koon were also charged with filing false reports. The trial of the four officers was moved from Los Angeles to Simi Valley in Ventura County.

On April 29, 1992, the jury handed down—except for one assault charge against Powell which ended in a hung jury—verdicts of not guilty on all counts. The acquittals touched off what became the most costly and destructive civil disturbance in this country in the 20th century. The disturbance began at the intersection of Florence and Normandy in the south central part of Los Angeles when rioters blocked traffic and beat dozens of motorists. Reginald Denny, a truck driver, was pulled out of his vehicle and beaten nearly to death. Looting began and buildings were set on fire.

As the violence grew, shop owners began defending their businesses with rifles. Los Angeles Mayor Tom Bradley requested that Governor Pete Wilson send in the National

Guard. Over ten thousand guardsmen were deployed to the streets of Los Angeles. A city-wide curfew was declared. By morning hundreds of fires were burning and at least a dozen people were dead. On May 1st, President George H. W. Bush ordered the 7th Infantry Division and the 1st Marine Division plus riot-trained federal officers to take control of the city.

The six days of unrest left fifty-eight people dead and approximately two thousand injured. Over eleven thousand people were arrested. Almost four thousand buildings were destroyed or damaged resulting in over one billion dollars in property damage.

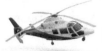 **IN THE AIR WITH JEFF!**

The 1992 Los Angeles riots began for me on that Wednesday afternoon with a Los Angeles Police Department (LAPD) radio dispatch that I monitored, for "an officer needs assistance call" not far from what would become ground zero of the unrest.

The dispatch stated that rocks and bottles were being thrown at officers by a large group. We were directly over Universal Studios, Universal City, when it hit. I asked the pilot if we could go to an area as close to Florence and Vermont as fast as possible. We got there in about four minutes.

What I saw was indeed an unusual event. A couple of LAPD patrol cars were in the middle of an intersection close to 68th and Budlong and there was indeed a group of about 20 civilians moving about quickly in a disorganized manner. Immediately a few more patrol cars arrived and then even more seemed to appear from all directions.

I was on the 2-way to our editors asking if they wanted to

go live with what I judged to be, at that point, something that was putting our listeners in harm's way. After that I found myself describing moment by moment the events that unfolded below me for the better part of some 70 plus hours, night and day, except for fuel stops, pilot changes, cat naps at the airport and fast food snacks.

The opening moments and hours that followed until around 4:00 the following Thursday morning seemed to me to last forever.

The next call we went to was just to the West a bit, to the intersection of Florence and Normandy. Motorists were now being stopped by a larger and separate crowd. A liquor store on the northeast corner was already being looted and people were running in all directions.

I remember my first concern was to keep people from driving into or near Florence and Normandy! It was the main focus of my reports but I also found myself describing what I now called a mob trying to stop drivers. I remember one car with a woman driving being stopped by 3 or 4 people. Her door was pulled open and a tug of war over control of the car started between the driver and crowd while the car continued to slowly roll. Finally those involved in this seemed to lose interest and the woman was spared. Those once directly involved in that incident now joined another group and what they did next will stay in our memories forever.

Right in the middle of Florence and Normandy the driver of a tanker rig was forcibly dragged from the cab of the truck to the pavement and savagely beaten. Now it seemed like a frenzy of destruction. If it wasn't for what I still believe was the miss fire of a weapon, Reginald Denny would have also been shot after the beating stopped!

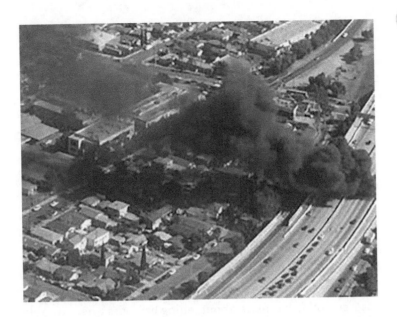

Around this time I remember our pilot relaying the word from LAPD Air Support that they believed they were being fired at from the ground and we should all be aware of the threat. In the air and on the ground below me this event was gaining in size, purpose and level of emergency faster than anything I had ever witnessed in airborne reporting.

As it happened that day we had some passengers in the back seat along for a ride—Los Angeles radio icon "Uncle Joe" Benson and his wife, Jan. Flying with guests on board was almost a daily occurrence prior to 9/11. At about 6:00 PM we had to go for fuel and concern of our passengers' safety and exposure to all this became critical so we headed back to Van Nuys Airport. After refueling we returned to the general area south of the Los Angeles Coliseum.

I remember using this phrase as I described what I was seeing, "From the air this looks like a cigarette hole in a napkin that very quickly is burning out in all directions." The words just tumbled out of my mouth.

The fires that were now burning in structures around the Harbor Freeway from Martin Luther King Jr. Boulevard towards Century Boulevard reminded me of the pictures that we had seen from the oil fires in Kuwaiti Oil Fires during Desert Storm. It was overpowering. Los Angeles Police Department radio dispatches came every few seconds alerting us to looting, fire, and beatings. It was endless.

I recall my editor saying to me that their news format was out the window now and that I was to monitor the station at all times. News anchors would just come to me without warning or lead with something like, "Jeff, what do you see now?"

That first night was way too soon for judgment or moral assessment. It was more about telling listeners where trouble was, where it seemed to be headed, and to be aware that an extraordinary event was taking place in our city that was picking up-tempo with every hour.

"Call family. Check in with grandparents. And make sure you know where your children are."

As the days and nights went by the Mayor, the Governor, and finally President Bush would become directly involved. The original "Officer needs help" near Florence and Normandy would grow like that "hole in the napkin" to most of South Los Angeles, Downtown Los Angeles, Korea town, Pico Robertson, Mid City and Hollywood.

I remember watching from the air an electronics store near Sunset and La Brea being looted and seeing a van that was so overloaded with stolen property it actually got hung up on a driveway and couldn't budge until some of the merchandise was taken out and just tossed to the ground. On into West Los Angeles it all continued with no sign of stopping. At one moment I remember pointing out to a freelance photographer who had joined us for a while in the back seat on Thursday what would have been a beautiful sunset, just barely getting through the smoke and soot of fires in Mid City Los Angeles.

It seemed from my vantage point that stores were being looted just for the sake of people getting caught up in the madness of it all. Certainly under daily circumstances people would never dream of such a thing but on it went. Eventually into Friday morning the effects of this outburst of anger and frustration was felt deep into the San Fernando Valley as far North as the LAPD Foothill Division on Osborne Street.

On Friday morning, although unrest was still going on, it appeared to me that all involved were just getting exhausted. The situation was starting to ebb and finally that afternoon around 6:00 I heard Ken Jeffries at KFWB say, "Jeff, I think you and your pilot can go home now!"

It's tough but I wish most people had turned to radio and television for more help and instruction. I think while being threatened by such dramatic events unfolding in your face, in might be hard to stop and ask for help or stop and plan some alternative action.

From the air I've watched some people just seem to shut down, to just sit there and do nothing! I'll forever wish Reginald Denny had heard our early reports and then had not made that left turn on Florence. I had the most amazing view of a major city unraveling before me, almost to a point of total destruction. I truly believe, be it a simple traffic event or a major disaster of some type, personal or otherwise, one must always have a plan, B, C and D and know where to turn for help. Do something positive. Going miles out of your normal way, to keep moving forward and get to where you need to be is so empowering.

 ON THE GROUND WITH MARY!

The events after the Rodney King verdict were rooted in decades of disenfranchisement, poverty, anger, and distrust. There is much to learn from that uprising and much to change to address its root causes. Many changes were made and many remain so deserving of attention. The causes of that unrest continue and the possibility for more disturbances lie in waiting beneath the surface of everyday life.

The metaphor I've chosen is in no way designed to avoid or denigrate those core issues. What I've tried to do is create a metaphor based on one particular behavior during that time of intense unrest and then apply it across the board to the broader range of human behavior.

During the riots people took items from stores for which they often had no need. This behavior during those times of unrest is called 'looting'. Looting might be a way to level the playing field or to get that which has been impossible to acquire. Looting might also possibly be an expression of fear or anger. During intense times, acquiring 'things' can help us feel heard, empowered, and perhaps even more safe.

Sometimes keeping those 'things' can also help us feel safe. During the days after the Rodney King verdict few people felt safe. Since fear is contagious, even people far removed from the uprisings exhibited behaviors associated with self-comforting.

The learning opportunity I've chosen has little to do with civil unrest and more to do with emotional unrest. Our need to acquire and keep 'things' can, if unchecked, become a significant issue.

At the time of this event, I lived about 20 miles from Florence and Normandy or in Los Angeles driving language about 30 minutes away. I knew about the events in South Central Los Angeles and I was worried about the people living in that area but I wasn't worried for my personal safety. After all, thirty minutes is a long way from the danger. However, I was out of paper towels and decided to go buy some.

When I got to the supermarket the first thing I noticed was that the parking lot was full. That was unusual considering the time of day and the day of the week. Inside, the place was utter chaos. People raced up and down the aisles just tossing things into their carts. They were stockpiling things that even under extreme circumstances they probably wouldn't need. For a few moments I considered joining the melee and tossing unnecessary items into my shopping cart too. But I paused, took a deep breath, bought my roll of paper towels and went home.

The stockpiling shoppers were frightened and when we experience fear our behavior can change. The challenge is to evaluate the fear and monitor our behavior.

Sometimes it's perfectly reasonable to make sure we've got sufficient supplies. In fact, we are often told to keep at least a three-day supply of water, food, medicines, and cash in case there's a massive disaster and we are on our own. Making sure we have these essential items will hopefully be accomplished in a calm, thoughtful, reasonable manner and in advance of any catastrophic event.

The shoppers I saw on the day the riots began were not by and large filling their shopping carts with essential items and they certainly weren't going about this in calm, thoughtful, reasonable manners.

Those were scary times in Los Angeles and many people felt the need to 'hoard' whether or not they needed the items in their carts. Hopefully when the fires were out and the danger passed those people stopped their frantic stockpiling.

Sometimes, though, even in normal circumstances we find it hard to let go of things. Keeping things or acquiring things can help us feel less anxious or frightened. And let's face it. Life can sometimes feel pretty scary. The challenge is to manage our fear, our anxiety, so that we don't start spending money and storage space on things for which we have no need either practically or emotionally.

We keep possessions because somehow in the keeping or in the acquiring we feel less anxious and a little safer. Up to a point that's okay. In fact, not only can hoarding be an important survival behavior, we aren't the only species doing it. Many different species, in order to survive long winters, stockpile or hoard food supplies. People living on the East Coast of this country, for example, sometimes use the behavior of squirrels to predict the severity of winter. If squirrels seem to be gathering a lot of food and carrying it into their nests people might say they are in for a long, cold winter.

So you see, hoarding can be a survival behavior. However, if your need to hang onto things is making your life more complicated than more enjoyable or easier, you might want to ask yourself whether or not you are becoming or already are a hoarder. This information doesn't mean you're bad or lazy but it might mean that you could benefit from a little help. It is estimated that about three million people in this country suffer from some degree of a hoarding disorder.

Here are some questions that can help you determine whether or not things are getting a little out of hand. Go ahead and answer them. Try to be objective. We're not looking over your shoulder. We won't see your answers. We just want to help make your travels a little easier. Put a check mark or an X in the circle next to the question if it applies to you even a little bit.

- I buy things knowing I don't need them or at least won't need them in the near future.
- My home is beginning to feel really cluttered. I don't have room to put away my stuff.
- If something is free I really want it. I've got all sorts of promotional item and I've got no use for any of them.
- I don't much want people to come into my home because the amount of clutter is embarrassing.

Thanks for answering those questions. Here's some space to write down your reactions to the questions. Just jot down whatever thoughts or feelings you experienced when you read and responded to them. Once again, there is no judgment here. Without information it's hard to make adjustments for easier travels.

....

....

....

....

....

Let's go a little further with this. Think of an item you've had for awhile but for which you have no use and which doesn't mean anything to you. If you have some of those 'give away' promotional items maybe choose one. Or maybe an old magazine or a T-shirt with too many holes to wear outside. Now think of that possession and try to answer these questions with yes or no.

1. If I throw this away I will feel really sad and I don't know why I'll feel that way. ....

....

2. I don't want to throw this away because I'm worried that I might need it at some point in the future.

....

3. I feel responsible for this possession and if I get rid of it I will feel like I shirked my responsibilities.

....

4. Someone else might need or want this and if I throw it away I won't be able to give it to that person.

....

5. I don't want anyone else to have this so I'm going to keep it. ....

....

Here's some space for you if you want to write down your reactions to those questions. Once again, this isn't about feeling guilty or stupid or any other negative emotion. It's about gathering useful information.

....

....

If you suspect that you are a 'hoarder' please don't start beating yourself up. There's nothing wrong with hanging onto 'stuff' unless your home is unhealthy or unsafe. However, not being able to clean up the clutter can make life more difficult. And even then what you are doing isn't necessarily wrong. All of your stuff, though, may be making it harder for you to get to where you want to be.

There were no right or wrong answers to those questions. We presented them to you so you could learn a little more about yourself. Remember that stockpiling or hoarding can be lifesaving. We react to actual or perceived dangers by doing things to help us feel safer. As long as they weren't stealing items or destroying property, those folks in the supermarket thirty minutes from the dangers of the Los Angeles riots were just trying to feel safe. It was an anxious time and they were just trying to feel a little less anxious.

Sometimes it's hard to change the behavior when the danger passes. Sometimes we hang on to our anxieties or fears for so long we almost forget the scary time happened. And yet we keep stockpiling and hoarding. That's why it's useful every once in awhile to check in with ourselves and see how we're doing.

Here are some useful check in questions:

I'm feeling anxious and unsafe. Am I in actual danger right now? (In order to answer this question it's necessary to take an objective assessment of your situation. Try to separate that assessment from your feelings.)

❑ Yes   ❑ No

If the answer is 'No' then take a deep breath and go on

about your business. Try to concentrate on your breathing and on the task at hand.

If the answer is 'Yes' ask yourself some more questions.

Am I in physical danger from the environment or from a living thing? In other words is this danger external?

❑ Yes   ❑ No

If the answer is 'Yes' take measures to get to safety. Those measures might include calling for assistance (911) or more extreme behaviors. In other words, do something to get yourself out of danger.

If your answer is 'No' then investigate further until you are satisfied of your safety.

We have a built in mechanism which helps us react to perceived or actual dangers. It's called the 'fight or flight' response. When we believe we are in danger our bodies, reacting to chemicals released by our brains, prepare us to either run for our lives or fight for our lives. You've probably experienced many of the physical manifestations of this response. These physical symptoms associated with the fight or flight response can range from uncomfortable to terrifying. They may manifest themselves as anxiety attacks or as indigestion or sore muscles. They may even take the form of panic attacks. Don't hesitate to seek medical attention for these symptoms.

The moment we believe we are in danger our brains start this life saving series of responses. Nerve cells fire and chemicals such as adrenaline, noradrenaline and cortisol are released into our bloodstream. These firings and releases create some intense changes in our bodies. Our respiratory rate increases resulting in faster and more shallow breathing. If we're going to fight for our lives or run for our lives there's no time to digest that meal we just ate. Blood is directed away from our digestive tracts and to our muscles. We need that extra fuel for the fight or the flight. We need to see as clearly as possible so our pupils may dilate. Our sensory awareness becomes sharper. Our reactions may quicken while our perception of events may slow down. This quickening and slowing may be a bit like the Major League batter whose senses are so keen he can see the seams on the ball heading toward him at 90 miles an hour. Our brains have prepared our bodies in a matter of seconds to respond mentally and physically to the danger.

We look around us for the saber toothed tiger. Unfortunately for this response mechanism, saber toothed tigers have been extinct for millions of years. And yet we still have this amazing response to danger. While it's true that even without saber toothed tigers we do encounter dangers, most of those dangers are more perceived than actual.

Without this innate fight or flight response, we as a species probably wouldn't have survived. This response was and continues to be designed for short term use so we can deal quickly with the threat in just a few minutes or seconds.

Even though our dangers today are vastly different from the days of the saber toothed tiger, the fight or flight response remains unchanged. Even though many of today's dangers are more psychological than physical they are often chronic. Concerns over saber toothed tigers have been replaced by financial, health, housing, justice, employment, retirement, relationship or equality concerns. Each time our health insurance challenges a prescription or each time our credit cards are maxed out we perceive a threat to our safety which releases the fight or flight response.

It seems that we now live in states of heightened alert and all too often we begin to consider everything in our environment as a possible threat to our survival. Back in prehistoric times our fight or flight response bypassed rational thought. There wasn't time to consider the age or the physical condition of our attacker. We reacted automatically without thought.

Except in cases of obvious emergency, we now have the luxury of time. We can think about our perceptions of danger. Taking the time to think things out, though, takes practice. We're not used to taking that time. However, since we are neither running or fighting for our lives, we do not discharge the chemicals released for those activities. Without that discharge, we may experience the long term effects of our fight or flight responses. We might experience medical problems. We might engage in negative coping mechanisms such as over eating, drinking too much, using drugs or even exercising so much that we do ourselves physical harm. One of those maladaptive coping mechanisms might be hoarding.

If we are physically safe and we know it, then our perception of not being safe is based on our thoughts. That's what was going on with most of the people in the supermarket the day the riots began. They listened to news reports and felt unsafe despite the fact that they were many miles and many minutes from the danger.

We can also feel unsafe or anxious because of events that happened long ago. We can worry that they will happen again. And so we do things to help us feel safer. It's really useful to develop the ability to evaluate our situations. It's also really useful to without judgment recognize the behaviors that help us feel safer. If those behaviors are ultimately complicating our lives, it's okay and necessary to modify those behaviors. Again, without judgment.

So, if you like to keep stuff and you rented a storage room because your home got too cluttered and you can afford the storage fee, go for it. However, if you never look at the contents of your storage room and yet you are considering renting another one because you've acquired more stuff you might consider getting rid of some of your possessions.

Getting rid of our possessions can be really difficult because, after all, we acquired and kept them to help us feel safe. You can lighten the load slowly. You can get help. Or you can keep it all until the day you die. Between now and then, though, you might ask yourself if there's something more enjoyable or productive you could be doing with the money spent on storage.

Once again, there's no judgment. We're just here to help you. And trust us. Making the load a little lighter can feel really good. Feeling really good is another way to feel safe.

SUICIDE ON A MAJOR TRANSITION

On May 1, 1998, Daniel V. Jones parked his pickup truck on the elevated ramp connecting the southbound Harbor Freeway (the 101) to the westbound Century Freeway (the 105). After a standoff lasting hours and witnessed by millions of television viewers as well as the hundreds stopped on the freeway below, Mr. Jones set fire to his truck and killed himself and Gladys, his black Labrador Retriever.

This event began as one of the many car chases for which Los Angeles streets and freeways are famous. It ended tragically in one of the most graphic events ever to develop on a Los Angeles freeway and in the process created miles-long traffic jams during the evening commutes.

Daniel V. Jones was a maintenance worker at a Long Beach hotel. He had worked at that hotel for over three years. He lived in a small bungalow practically hidden by a tall, wooden fence bearing a 'Beware of Dog' sign. A few weeks before his death, Mr. Jones had been, according to a neighbor, diagnosed as having a cancerous growth on his neck. He also told the neighbor that he was 'getting the run around' from his Health Maintenance Organization (HMO). His sister later disclosed that Mr. Jones recently learned that he was HIV+ and was also frustrated by the HMO's apparent reluctance to cover that medical condition.

When Mr. Jones parked his pickup on the elevated transition loop, motorists began calling emergency numbers reporting that a man, with a dog sitting beside him, was pointing a shotgun at passing cars. Authorities immediately closed both the Harbor Freeway and the Century Freeway. Traffic stopped in all directions.

Mr. Jones called 911 and spoke to California Highway Patrol Dispatcher Lieutenant Hanns Ruth.

"He was just rambling. He mentioned he was unhappy about HMOs."

While talking to Lt. Ruth, Mr. Jones fired several rounds from the shotgun. One went through the pickup's roof. He remained in the truck while police helicopters flew overhead and the Los Angeles County Sheriff's Special Weapons Team assembled nearby.

Eventually Mr. Jones got out of his pickup, reached back in and pulled out what looked to be a backpack. He started taking clothing out of it and then a videocassette tape. He then threw the backpack and its contents over the wall onto the empty Harbor Freeway below. He next unfurled a large banner and hung it from the railing. The hand-lettering read: "HMO's are in it for the money!! Live free, love safe or die." After making a few obscene gestures he returned to his pickup, got in, petted Gladys, and sipped from a beverage can.

Just as SWAT team negotiators were about to begin trying to persuade him to give up, the truck burst into flames. He had made several Molotov cocktails. They were in the cab of the pickup and, according to Los Angeles Police Lieutenant Anthony Alba, he deliberately lit at least one.

His clothes on fire and in obvious pain, Mr. Jones jumped out of his vehicle frantically trying to pat out the flames. He was able to take off his pants, shoes, socks, and underwear. Naked from the waist down, he staggered to the railing gesturing angrily. It appeared that he was about to jump. Instead of jumping, though, he backed away from the railing, staggered to his pickup, got his shotgun, placed the barrel beneath his chin, and pulled the trigger. He died instantly. Gladys died in the burning pickup.

Law enforcement, fearing more explosives in the pickup, waited some time to approach the area. Once they did they discovered more Molotov cocktails, several shotgun shells and exploded containers of gasoline and propane.

The 105 and the 110 freeways remained closed for several more hours backing traffic up more than five miles. The charred cement sides of the transition ramp could be seen for well over a year.

 IN THE AIR WITH JEFF!

For most of my years at KFWB News 98, I was on standby 24 hours a day. What that meant was that KFWB or Shadow/Metro could call or page me and I was expected to get to Van Nuys Airport ASAP. Through the years it happened quite a bit, but I enjoyed the commitment and the adventure of it all. This page came at a time when I was on my way to the Airport for the afternoon shift that usually started at 3:50. The newsroom said a short pursuit had ended at the 110/105 Interchange and was turning into a standoff with police. I think we were airborne and on the way by 3:20 or so. Upon arriving my first assessment to the newsroom, off the air, was that this was a bit different from the average "End of Pursuit" car chase standoff.

The location where the individual had come to a stop was at the apex of the transition from the southbound Harbor 110 Freeway to the westbound Century Freeway towards Los Angeles International Airport. It was a bit before 4:00 PM and the hard-core afternoon rush had begun at this crucial interchange in Los Angeles. The driver was armed with what reporting motorists described as a shotgun. He was not alone. A medium size dog was in the cab and the pickup truck was, as far as police, were concerned, still drivable. This meant that the suspect could get back in and make the threat mobile again.

We arrived and set up some slow orbits around the interchange. My first reports on the air described briefly what was happening. I could plainly see the man who was quite agitated and armed with a short-barreled weapon of some type. I thought it was probably a shotgun. He continued to get in and out of the pickup. I could see the dog in the cab. Then the man unfurled a bed sheet type banner that said something about HMO's or health care. The situation was ramping up very fast and the suspect was moving around a lot.

After the first few on-air reports I started to focus on the traffic implications, which were escalating rapidly. The 110 freeway was now closed in both directions leading to and under the 105 freeway. The still new 105 was closed in both directions going over the 110. The big problem and what would become THE story was getting to LAX. It was becoming difficult and would soon be impossible to get to the airport from many directions. One of the big reasons for building the Century freeway (105) was that it would run in-between the 605 freeway and the airport (LAX). This simplified life for drivers of motor vehicles as well as the Green Line Light Rail system. It turned that freeway into a major lifeline.

Now that lifeline was closed and so was the connector from the 110 freeway. These two freeways and their connectors handled an enormous volume of evening traffic leaving downtown Los Angeles.

As far as the evening traffic was concerned, everything was squaring itself to "infinity and beyond!" More police arrived. This event had become a multi-jurisdiction affair because of the location. The Los Angeles Police Department, the California Highway Patrol, the Los Angeles County Sheriff Department, and the Los Angeles County and City Fire Departments were all involved. Crews and more crews kept arriving to the scene.

We were not alone in the air. There were other media helicopters as well as law enforcement helicopters. Pilots had to avoid each other, give Police Air Support lots of room to work, and also talk with LAX air controllers and Hawthorne Airport controllers as well as talk to arriving and departing aircraft to both locations. Everyone involved was focused and aware.

Below me thousands of motorists were also involved in the tragedy. They no doubt had strong thoughts and feelings about the events on the transition ramp. They also had other thoughts and feelings: I must catch my plane. I've got to get to work. I'm late for my child's reunion gate at school. I'm frantic because I've got to get to my child's day care.

I was in the "This is what's going on here but this is what you must do to avoid this extraordinary situation," mode!

There were lots of drivers just caught in the middle of it all sitting on roads and freeways. They were stopped with their engines off. They were stuck and beyond frustrated! Drivers were calling newsrooms demanding help and answers. We were hearing from calls made by our newsrooms to LAX that some flights were leaving almost empty so many people were missing their planes!

As I was thinking this was just out of control, it got much worse. The man set himself on fire and then probably changed his mind because he was out of the truck tearing off his clothes. He was clearly suffering. Sadly, his dog had already succumbed to the fire. I thought he was going to jump from the overpass but then events spiraled down so fast. The man ended his life by using the weapon he had brandished through this whole event.

All of this played out live on radio and television including the fatal gunshot. That afternoon ultimately led to changes in television coverage of such events. The goal of those changes was to never again show on television news such things to the unsuspecting viewer.

This story, though, was far from over. Police, justifiably, had procedures to follow with this type of event. They couldn't be sure that the area was safe and secure. The possibility of booby traps or other possible injury causing devices could still be aboard the truck.

It wasn't until around 7:00 in the evening that the interchange was opened. The police investigation ran late into the night. The actions of one person had cost unimaginable sudden change to thousands and thousands of people that day. The events left police and others working into the night. They turned a major international airport upside down and left many a child tearfully waiting to go home.

 ON THE GROUND WITH MARY!

The public suicide of Daniel V. Jones was dramatic beyond description. The fact that his dog also died seemed to intensify the tragedy. Millions of people either directly or indirectly witnessed his death. Had Mr. Jones stayed in his bungalow and killed himself in quiet privacy his death would doubtless have gone unnoticed except for family, friends, and co-workers. However, his death would have placed him without incident among the 30,000 people in this country who kill themselves each year.

There are people right now reading this book who are seriously thinking about suicide. Some of you may have actually tried to commit suicide. Many others reading this page have a close friend or a loved one who has attempted or committed suicide.

In this country, right now, suicide is considered to be a major medical problem. That number of 30,000 annual deaths by suicide hasn't gone down over the past thirty years. In fact, the number is now rising steadily because of military related suicides.

In 1999 Dr. David Stacher, then Surgeon General of the United States, proposed a national plan to serve as a roadmap toward developing a comprehensive national suicide prevention strategy. The key features of the plan became the acronym AIM (Awareness, Intervention and Methodology) to define what he believed would be the relevant components of a national strategy. He hoped to make suicide a public health issue, which would require support and direction from the federal government. The plan was sidetracked by the events of 9/11 and has yet to get back on track.

Obviously the primary cost of this major medical problem is loss of life. However, suicide also significantly impacts the nation's work force. Our most recent information indicates that lost productivity due to suicide is over eleven billion dollars a year. Tragically, employed adults aren't the only people killing themselves. Suicide is the third leading cause of death for children ages ten to fourteen years of age.

The most common method of suicide (over 56%) is from self-inflicted gunshot wounds. In one year attempted suicides resulted in 700,000 emergency room visits of which 152,000 were admitted because of the severity of the attempt.

My career as a social worker has focused primarily on helping suicidal children and adults buy some time in which to stay alive and in which to hopefully find reasons to live or to learn more effective ways of coping with their anger or pain or disappointment. My attempts at buying time haven't always been successful. When someone I'm trying to help succeeds at suicide, those left behind have one primary question on their minds and in their hearts. Those left behind want to know why.

Why are we killing ourselves or trying to kill ourselves at such alarming rates? From my decades of helping suicidal adults and children buy time I have come to the conclusion that we feel suicidal when we perceive a loss of empowerment. We think of killing ourselves when suicide is the only voice we feel we have. We have no control over anything else but we can control whether we live or die and when we die.

We all need to feel that we have a say in how we live our lives. We also need to believe that we can be successful in specific situations with specific tasks. At a very early age, babies need to know they can perform tasks even if the task is grasping the finger of the primary caregiver. Self-confidence is built on our earliest accomplishments. Psychologist Albert Bandura coined the phrase self-efficacy and wrote about the major role it plays in how we approach goals, tasks, and challenges. A variety of scales have been developed to measure our self-efficacy. Those scales invite participants to rate statements such as:

1. I am always able to handle difficult situations.
2. I stay calm when confronting difficulties.
3. I use positive, good coping tools.

Such instruments can be useful for research or evaluation but I believe we know when we feel confident and when we don't. I also think we know when we feel angry or hopeless. Research indicates that depression is associated with suicide. I think that before the depression comes anger. I also believe that in our society we do not easily talk about feelings of anger or depression and we certainly don't comfortably talk about thoughts of suicide. That's a shame because those three subjects cry out for discussion.

Anger can be scary—scary to feel, scary to witness, and scary to express. I believe we need to learn more acceptable, healthy ways to express our anger. If we don't express anger in healthy ways, we may risk expressing it unhealthily and even illegally. We also risk sinking into depression. My experience leads me to believe that a large part of depression is unexpressed anger. Depression can leave us feeling powerless to have any type of control over our lives except whether we live or die.

I mentioned earlier that my only suicidal intervention is to help the person in distress buy some time in which to discover hope or passions or coping tools. I say that because whether someone ultimately chooses to live or to die is beyond my control. That may sound harsh but it is true.

There are many ways to help the person buy time. One method available to law enforcement and mental health professionals is involuntary psychiatric hospitalization. The original intention of involuntary hospitalization was to eliminate incarceration into mental asylums based on medical (and all too often family) determinations. Often these incarcerations were without set time limits. Thus arose the fear of being 'locked away forever' if I tell you that I'm thinking of killing myself. Indeed, up until the middle of the twentieth century many psychiatric hospitals were pretty awful places. On July 3, 1946, though, President Harry Truman signed the National Mental Health Act. Because of this law, the National Institute of Mental Health was created and psychiatric hospitals got better because of increased public awareness and increased oversight.

There remains, however, a stigma on mental illness. Because of this stigma, men, women, and children avoid seeking help. All too often the symptoms of mental illness become so severe that men and women enter the judicial system and are incarcerated not in the old mental institutions but in jails and prisons. The largest psychiatric facility in this country is the Los Angeles County Jail.

Because of the stigma of mental illness people thinking of suicide don't want to seek help for fear of being labeled 'crazy'. And so the anger and the depression continue and 30,000 people plus now a staggering number of veterans continue to kill themselves each year.

If you are thinking of killing yourself, please get help. Here are some referrals you can use **RIGHT NOW!**

- Call the Suicide Prevention Lifeline: 1-800-273-TALK (8255)
- Text CONNECT to 74141 from anywhere in the USA, anytime, about any type of crisis.

- Visit Suicide Prevention Services of America at http://www.spsamerica.org/

Talk to someone. Tell someone that you are considering suicide. Yes, it's true that you may be hospitalized against your will. I have hospitalized hundreds of suicidal men, women and children. While a few of those hospitalizations were voluntary, most weren't.

Today all fifty states plus the District of Columbia have civil commitment statutes requiring a determination of dangerousness because of a mental illness. That means that a mental health professional or a law enforcement officer must determine that a person is in danger of suicide. Even though the statutes do include mental illness, please don't let that stop you from seeking help. Mental illness covers such a broad spectrum of thoughts and feelings and behaviors that on any given day we would all meet some criteria and be determined mentally ill. Please, please. If you are thinking about killing yourself seek help from a hospital, from law enforcement, from your church, mosque or synagogue. Your life is much more important than what others may think about you.

The reason mental illness is included as criteria for involuntary hospitalization due to suicidal thoughts may seem a bit convoluted but it involves a United States Supreme Court ruling. In the 1975 case of *O'Connor v. Donaldson* the Court held that "A finding of 'mental illness' alone cannot justify locking up a person against his/her will and keeping him/her indefinitely in custodial confinement." What that decision means, I believe, is that someone cannot be 'locked up' just because of a mental illness nor can that same person be 'locked up' only because of a suicide intent and plan. That ruling placed a checks and balance system on involuntary hospitalization.

It's all very complicated and, quite frankly, the jury is still out about whether or not in the long run involuntary hospitalization helps keep a person alive. Here's what I do know, though. Hospitalization buys time.

There are many other ways to buy time. If you are thinking of killing yourself, please talk to someone. If you don't want to seek professional help, talk to a friend or a member of the clergy. Talk to the stranger on the suicide hot line. Please don't keep silent. Silence is so powerful and rarely helpful.

If someone comes to you disclosing thoughts of suicide, listen. Please listen without judgment. Listen without trying to fix the situation or banish the thoughts. Just listen. Listening is an amazingly powerful tool.

If you are worried that someone is thinking of suicide, please encourage discussion.

You might say something like, "I'm worried about you. I'm afraid you're thinking of killing yourself. Would you like to talk to me?"

Asking someone if they are thinking of suicide is not going to cause a suicide attempt. It may, however, help the person feel heard and it might help the person regain a sense of self-efficacy.

Listening to someone's thoughts of suicide is not about keeping secrets. If the person's plans are immediate, you can save a life by calling '911'. Yes, the suicidal person may be angry with you. Many people I've hospitalized have been angry with me. The point is not to make friends but to save a life by buying the person time.

With time we might develop sufficient self-efficacy to approach our problems with more confidence. With time we might remember that life is ultimately worth living.

With time we might remember that none of us will survive this life. We are all going to die someday. Knowing that, we might choose to embrace the time we have and ultimately be thankful that someone helped us buy some more time.

Research indicates that having a sense of belonging and being comfortable with seeking help contribute to decreased thoughts of suicide. Despite the Surgeon General's 1999 Call To Action, it's apparent that the public health community has not fully embraced suicide prevention and continues to focus on treatment for the suicidal person. I believe that we need to shift our focus to prevention. We do that by finding meaning in our own lives and helping others find meaning in their lives.

Talk to someone. Listen to someone without judgment. Reclaim your voice. Help others do the same.

I don't know that having someone to talk to would have saved the life of Daniel V. Jones. Perhaps he needed more help than that. I do know, though, that no one should ever have to reach the point of such desperation and powerlessness that they feel their only choice is to die.

I can at least begin with taking good care of my physical and emotional self. You can do the same. I can at least reach out to you and ask if you are okay. You can do the same for me. Together, I believe we can slow down this epidemic called suicide.

THE NORTHRIDGE EARTHQUAKE >>

The thing about natural disasters is that they happen. We can't keep them from happening and we can't stop them once they start. Tornados, hurricanes, and earthquakes rip apart lives. We can prepare for them. We can build cellars. We can secure furniture and appliances to the walls. Once the storms hit or once the ground begins to shake, though, we run or hang on for our lives. That's the way it is with natural disasters.

Sometimes we get warning. Sometimes we get absolutely no warning. People who live in what we call 'earthquake country' often create predictors. Birds fly away. Dogs bark. Certain weather characteristics are called earthquake weather. I suspect we create those predictors to help us feel that we have some control over events. We like to have control. However, natural disasters leave us feeling helpless. We are neither in control nor are we in charge.

On January 17, 1994, at 4:30:55 AM PST a magnitude 6.7 earthquake, with its epicenter in the Los Angeles suburb of Reseda, hit. The actual, initial, violent shaking lasted about twenty seconds even though everyone who felt it would swear that initial shaking lasted about twenty years. The ground acceleration produced by the earthquake was the highest ever recorded in an urban area of this continent. It shook Las Vegas, Nevada—220 miles from the Reseda epicenter. About a minute after that initial seismic event an aftershock of magnitude 6.0 rattled nerves and structures already strained to capacity. Eleven hours later, just as residents began to trust the earth again, another 6.0 aftershock hit. Thousands of aftershocks continued for months and devastated already damaged buildings, trapping many people below the rubble of parking structures and freeway overpasses.

It is generally hard if not impossible to determine the exact number of deaths and injuries directly caused by a natural disaster. People die of indirect causes such as heart attacks and these deaths can happen months after the actual event. The official counts seem to agree, though, that fifty-seven people were killed in the immediate earthquake, more than 8,700 were injured including 1,600 requiring hospitalization, 20,000 were left homeless and more than 40,000 buildings were damaged in Los Angeles, Ventura, Orange and San Bernardino Counties. The earthquake permanently raised the ground 20 inches in various parts of the San Fernando Valley. Damage was recorded as far away as 52 miles from the heart of the shake.

Eleven hospitals suffered structural damage and had to transfer their patients to other facilities. Structural damage was reported to more than 12,000 homes, businesses, schools and hospitals, leaving many people homeless for extended periods.

The Los Angeles Memorial Coliseum, home to the 1932 and 1984 Olympics, suffered more than $44 million in damage. Farther south of downtown, the Watts Towers sustained $2 million damage that required seven years to repair. California State University-Northridge sustained significant damage. In the three years that followed the Northridge Earthquake, more than 681,000 residents applied for assistance from federal and state governments—making the earthquake both a devastating natural and economic disaster.

California is famous not only for its earthquakes also for its earthquake fault lines of which about 250 are known. The most famous fault is the San Andreas. In fact, the San Andreas Fault line may be the most famous earthquake fault in the world. It's over 800 miles long. That's almost 65% of the length of the state.

You'd think that every earthquake in the state would be somewhere on this fault line. That's not the case, though. In fact, the Northridge Earthquake occurred on a previously undiscovered fault. Now it has a name: The Northridge Blind Thrust Fault.

The Northridge Meadows apartment complex was one of the best-known affected buildings. When it collapsed sixteen people died. Throughout the greater Los Angeles area parking structures collapsed like houses of cards. In all, eight Southern California freeways were damaged, including the Highway 14 and Interstate 5 interchange. The interchange's collapse cut off freeway access to Los Angeles for hundreds of thousands of residents of northern Los Angeles County. The vast and famous Los Angeles freeway network serves millions of commuters every day. Damage to the Santa Monica Freeway, Interstate 10, one of the busiest freeways in the United States, congested nearby surface roads for months while the freeway was repaired.

Los Angeles Police Department motorcycle officer Clarence Wayne Dean died when he fell 40 feet from the collapsed Newhall Pass interchange connecting the southbound 14 to southbound I-5. Because of the early morning darkness, he couldn't see that the elevated roadway no longer existed. When the interchange was rebuilt again one year later, it was renamed the Clarence Wayne Dean Memorial Interchange in his honor.

Broken gas lines from houses shifting off their foundations or from unsecured water heaters falling over caused widespread fires. In the San Fernando Valley, several underground gas and water lines ruptured. Many streets had simultaneous fires and floods going on. In some neighborhoods water pressure dropped to zero, which made fire hydrants practically useless. Days after the earthquake approximately 60,000 households were still without public water service.

An interesting after effect of the Northridge earthquake was an outbreak of coccidioidomycosis (Valley Fever) in Ventura County. This is a respiratory disease caused by inhaling airborne fungus spores. In an eight-week period after the earthquake, 203 cases were reported. Three people who sought medical treatment for Valley Fever during that time died. The 203 three cases were about 10 times the normal rate in an 8-week period. It was also the first report of a Valley Fever outbreak following an earthquake. Earthquakes can stir up a lot of dust especially if they cause landslides. Since just about everything in Southern California can cause a landslide or a mudslide, it was inevitable that the Northridge Earthquake caused seismically triggered landslides, which resulted in large clouds of dust. Most of the Valley Fever cases were in folks who lived immediately downwind from those landslides. The natural conclusion was that the blowing dust carried those fungus spores right into people's lungs. Those who contracted and/or died of Valley Fever were not counted among the injured or deceased.

The ripple damage of natural disasters (or any catastrophic event for that matter) is all too often simply impossible to estimate. In one way or another we are all impacted to some degree. Natural disasters are ranked. We like to know the score of things and where we stand, it seems. The rankings are generally determined not by the number of lives lost but by the dollar amount of damage done. Based on that ranking rationale, the Northridge Earthquake continues to be one of the most expensive natural disasters in world history.

It's easy to find lists of world disasters which calculate the cost of damage based on inflation or today's replacement costs. Those lists may also indicate not only the cost of natural disasters financially but the lives lost. Clearly, some of the most devastating disasters in lost lives were not that costly in damage. However, no dollar sign can be put on lost lives. Nor can a dollar sign be put on emotional distress. Years after the winds have stopped blowing or the waters have receded or the earth has stopped shaking the people who were there and the first responders who got there continue to experience the long-lasting impacts of physical, emotional, cognitive and spiritual trauma.

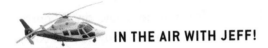 **IN THE AIR WITH JEFF!**

The buzzer goes off and I somehow pull myself into semi-consciousness from that mystical, non-sensible state of dreaming or not dreaming. I hit the alarm button and swing my feet from the bed to the floor and then just sit there for a moment wondering.

"How do I do this day after day after day?"

So for me, it's shuffle off the kitchen, hit the brew button and start the routine: Make the bed. Hit the head. Get the eyeballs focused. Look at the man in the mirror for a few seconds. Shake my head in disbelief. Stumble back to the kitchen for COFFEE! This has been my daily routine for more than 25 years. Monday through Friday my day begins at 3:35 in the morning.

Sometimes the paper comes early and is at my door. For me this is a giant plus in case there is a continuing story like a brush fire or something that goes on for a few days. It's good to read the print version to see if I got it right while I was reporting live and perhaps look at maps of the region involved. So far today is my lucky day. The paper is on the doormat. Welcome! So, coffee and paper in hand I sit at the dining room table and try to move into consciousness.

All is as it should be for about a half an hour and then something happened that I had never experienced before and hope to never again. I originally thought it weird that the room, everything in it including me, was starting to sway ever so gently. It was instant nausea time but I didn't get the luxury of time to be sick because in just a few seconds this weird moment ramped up to terror, confusion and fear of the unknown that lasted another 30 to 45 seconds!

It was the sound that really got to me—some kind of horror movie groan that grew rapidly to deafening levels. The coffee cup was gone. The kitchen was behind me so I slowly turned to stand, forgetting all that media stuff about duck, cover and hold! As I turned the roar of the freight train reached my home and it was loud!

I'm hanging onto the counter for dear life and screaming out loud, "Stop it. Stop!"

It didn't stop, of course and now I'm watching the kitchen cabinets empty themselves onto the kitchen floor from both sides. The fridge opens and out comes everything in it. My stuff is flying every which way--pots, pans the toaster. The Sparkletts water dispenser goes over and all the water goes everywhere. Glasses I hadn't used for years tumble to the floor and turn into a maze of shrapnel.

I'm still yelling, "STOP!!!"

It didn't! I'm still hanging onto the counter. It seems like I'm frozen. I hear what had to be the TV take a death plunge in the living room. Something I can't quite make out goes across my field of vision from the hallway in-between the bedrooms and into the living room and then, oh joy, the lights go out!

Fear has turned into rage and I keep yelling, "Stop it!!!"

Finally it did. From this loud, horrible noise, a noise now burned into my memory chip forever, and the chaos of un-controlled movement that came with it, now suddenly there is silence. It took a few seconds to catch my breath but slowly I got it together and realized that I had just survived a pow-erful earthquake. As far as moments in my life rank that mo-ment of realization ranks right up there in the top 2 or 3. After about a minute I started to hear sounds that I could identify. People. Voices. My neighbors were shouting for help!

Thankfully I wasn't standing barefoot in the kitchen when I heard the calls for help because I would have been in the middle of a minefield of broken glass. Off to my bedroom I go cautiously for jeans, shoes and a sweatshirt and reality. My place is a mess. My place is an apartment in what was once called North Hollywood but now "gentrified" to Valley Village. It was built in the 1960s. It's a 2-story garden apart-ment style building still owned by the original owner's fam-ily. It was a Los Angeles gem. Everyone loved it. Now, though, it was a mess. More on that later.

Once dressed, I grab a flashlight (so prepared!!) and go outside to check on friends and neighbors. There is a lot of chatter and talk going on but no one is trapped or hurt! That's quite a miracle considering the entire rear part of the building has dropped about 2 feet but is somehow still standing.

Everyone I can care for is okay so my next thought is, "I need to get to the airport."

Understand that I didn't need to get to the airport to get out of town but to go to work. The next hour went by quickly as one unexpected event after another unfolded before me.

First, as I left my apartment, I realized for the first time that I couldn't close the front door. It was partially off the hinges. My neighbor told me she wasn't leaving unless told to and would try to keep an eye on things. Next, I go to the rear of the building to the carport area and discover that area is partially collapsed. My car seems okay but I can't get it out and onto the street. I go back to the front of the building, which has become the gathering place for everyone. I join the gathering. Surprisingly, we all seem to be okay but I still can't get to the airport.

All of a sudden a Jeep pulls up in front of the building! This would ordinarily be a perfectly normal event but under the circumstances I found it to be extraordinary! It was like your dragon showing up to take you away. Roy Rodgers whistled for Trigger and he came galloping up! Wow!

The driver of the Jeep was a young man coming to take my neighbor's daughter to Northridge. She wanted to stay with her mother so I immediately asked him if he would take me to Van Nuys Airport.

With no hesitation whatsoever he said, "Let's go!"

We both hop into his Jeep and off we go. A major earthquake has hit early morning Los Angeles and I'm off to the airport in perhaps the perfect go through anything vehicle—a Jeep! How does this happen?

How is it that I have this "got to get to the airport and get to work" mentality? Maybe the D.I.'s at Parris Island knew what they were doing all along! Huh! Once a Marine always a Marine I guess. All the reasons to not move from home are there but I wanted to get to my job! Later on I'll discover that there were a lot of people with that same mentality and purpose. Meanwhile back in the Jeep, we're barreling west on the Ventura freeway towards Van Nuys. The two of us lean inches forward in our seats towards the windshield straining to see the roadway before us—like that would help! Too funny!!

All the roadways are intact and we make the Vanowen entrance to the South East corner of Van Nuys Airport seemingly in minutes only to meet a few others standing at the security gate. It's closed and our card keys won't work. Reality hits big time. I knew that power outages were occurring all over but surely that wouldn't stop me from getting to the airport, would it? Oh yeah it would and a lot of other people are experiencing similar issues. Talk about unexpected roadblocks in your life suddenly thrown at you!

My radio station, KFWB News 98, is on the air. The morning crew was already in the studio before the quake hit and reporters are checking in on 2-way radios. Some phone service is up but sporadic. Thanks to great engineers and solid planning KFWB and crew stay on the air. At the moment I took it for granted but days later I realized how extraordinary that would turn out to be. It was time for the little almost forgotten transistor radio to make a huge comeback. With power outages hitting all over Los Angeles television stations were out! Radios carried the information load—News Radio! People who weren't driving and listening sat in their parked cars or driveways listening to radio!

I would hear from listeners years later things like, "Boy, during the earthquake, you guys were all we had. Thanks!"

Meanwhile back to the gate at Van Nuys airport. We were all wondering how we were going to get in and once in would our hangar still be standing, was our helicopter crushed in the rubble and always why was there no one else here? Finally some of the night crew at Sky Trails, a fuel company at the airport, pulled up from the airport side of the fence. They, of course, were beyond stressed out due to all the calls from the FBO's on the field. The mood was quite chaotic all around. Of course the gate was powered by an electric motor with access controlled by electricity. We couldn't locate the override switch so the gate wouldn't budge. Some new comers to our little "Let Us In" party left to check on other gates around the field. I didn't expect them to have much luck since all of the gates were electronic. I stayed where I was and gave the fence a good, hard look. It didn't look like a friendly come climb me type of fence but I grew up in Brooklyn, New York. Over the fence I climbed. A few others climbed over, too. The only lights were from flashlights.

The Sky Trails guys had gone off to answer a few hundred calls for help so I started walking to the hangar. When I finally got there I was astonished to see that the hangar was still a hangar! It was still standing and appeared to be intact. I opened the locks and started pushing the massive doors out of the way. The hangar housed a P-51 Mustang, a 172 Cessna, 3 flight ready Bell Jet Rangers of different designations plus the usual extra parts, mechanics' tools, equipment and so on. Still clutching the flashlight from my home, I swept the beam across the hangar and really couldn't believe what I saw! Except for shelves and leaning stuff against walls now down, it looked pretty good. The most obvious damage was that none of the florescent light fixtures hanging from the ceiling had light tubes. The fluorescent tubes were broken and scattered all over most of the aircraft. They looked like they had been in a blizzard of glass.

"Wow, this is great," I thought and may have actually said aloud.

I had expected to find everything in a collapsed mess and was relieved to discover that things weren't that bad. I immediately started removing the big pieces from the aircraft and moved on to the smaller stuff. I also started calling owners, pilots, the radio station—everyone I knew. My cell phone worked and I wanted to make those calls while I had service. It was now about 5:20 in the morning. Less than two hours had passed since I had tried to drink my morning coffee!

KFWB was flooded with activity and every time I called the response was, "Please, get up in the air!"

Some pilots by now were returning my calls. Most were understandably more concerned with taking care of their families than with getting me up in the air. Quite frankly getting up in the air and helping people get where they want to go is about all I've got going for me so during those moments I had kind of a hard time understanding the reaction of the pilots. Looking back now, I wish I had had a family to look after, too.

I finally heard from Kevin LaRosa, Sr., the owner of Jet Copters. Kevin lived in the West Hills area and had finally managed to get his home security gate open. He was on his way to the airport! This was great news for me. Kevin had other contracts besides KFWBs' Jet Copter 98 and he wanted to get all the news media and networks in the air as soon as possible. On a personal level I was feeling anxious about what I was going to see once I was in the air. After what seemed like forever but was really only minutes Kevin arrived and put everything in motion. Calls, orders, wishes, pleas to pilots to get here ASAP! Since I was there staring at him, his first choice was easy. Fly me around until other pilots arrived and then tend to his other clients. After an overly cautious preflight we were flying! First thing for me was a quick check in with the KFWB desk and editors via the 2-way.

Yet another mini miracle happened when they replied, "Yeah we copy. Where are you?"

Wow. We're working. We're in the air. I took a deep breath and looked around the early morning darkness of the San Fernando Valley. The view was extraordinary. Kevin took off to the north. As we climbed I asked him to head towards the 118 Freeway and Granada Hills. My view from the left front seat was about 270 degrees and was filled with darkness, smatterings of light, a sliver of moon and exploding electrical transformers. Wherever I looked, the phosphorous trails of sparks and weirdly colored smoke from poles filled the San Fernando valley with explosions of light followed by darkness. Then I saw something more troubling than those light explosions. There were fires—a lot of fires.

I was now on the air live with KFWB. Pete Demetrio was also reporting live from his news van. The studio anchors were fielding hundreds of calls from everywhere.

Once again—like during the Los Angeles Riots of 1992—the editors said, "Just keep monitoring the station. We'll come to you unannounced. Be ready to go live at all times!"

I asked Kevin to get us over the largest fire just east of the I-5 and North of the 210 in Sylmar. It turned out to be a large mobile home park that seemed to have many small fires trying to merge as one big one. I remember saying that I thought it could have been a situation where the mobile homes were knocked off their foundations, splitting the gas lines and fire was just jumping from lot to lot. Even this early and barely two hours after the first jolts, at least three quarters of that area was fully consumed with flame. I could see a lot of movement on the ground—people running, cars moving and some first responders' emergency lights. As I'm describing this situation we make a sudden turn to the west. I'm stunned to see another large area of flame going straight up with great force. I don't even have to ask Kevin to go there. Our minds seem somehow connected and we are functioning almost as one person. He gently guides the helicopter to Balboa Boulevard near Rinaldi Street in Granada Hills. I keep looking at something but for the first couple of minutes can't figure it out at all. First, there is a wall of water rushing down south on Balboa towards the 118 but it's on fire! We later learned that a large gas main had broken and caught fire. A home in its path was practically incinerated. I suddenly realized that we were in an unusual spot for complete disaster. The enormous Los Angeles Reservoir was just uphill from all this. This was the very place where Mr. Mulholland and company brought water into the San Fernando Valley many years before. From this spot to Long Beach was all downhill—fifty miles of homes, oil refineries, businesses and lives! Thankfully the reservoir remained intact although there were some smaller failures. A river of water on fire. I'll never forget that one.

Wherever I look I see overwhelming chaos. My job, though, is to help people get to where they want to be as safely as possible. My job is to interpret my observations to my listeners.

"If you're here, do this. Don't go there. Call your parents. Check on your grandparents. This street is blocked. Stay home. Don't get on these roads. If you're driving, look out for this. If you're home, stay there."

It just didn't stop. I felt like I was talking to my own family. I so desperately wanted my listeners be safe that the words just rolled out of my mouth!

One of the most dramatic events began when a KFWB editor got on the 2-way and told me that the Newhall Pass was collapsing! The Newhall Pass, for those of you who have never been to Los Angeles, is a major interchange in the north end of the San Fernando Valley where two freeways merge or split depending on your direction. In the morning this pass brings thousands of commuters from the Antelope valley and Santa Clarita south into Los Angeles. It's made up of many roadways built over one another some 80 feet high finally leading to one road surface. This was a massive interchange, a lot of structure here. We were close by so north we went. As we flew through the pass I kept looking for the collapsed area. At first I didn't notice anything even though we were into daylight. All I mentally registered was the fact that there was no traffic coming south on the 14. It was stopping around what was then called San Fernando Road but which is now Newhall Avenue. We kept heading northeast until Kevin turned us back south towards the merge of the 14 and I-5. My mouth just fell open. We must have flown right over it coming through from the Valley side but there it was. I will never forget this most extraordinary view: Two massive failures—a section of the 14 just north of the interchange and a section of the I-5 north of the interchange! Two gaping, long stretches of the elevated sections lay on ground leaving vehicles stranded on one side or the other. One person died because of this collapse. Los Angeles Police Department Motor Officer Clarence Wayne Dean was rushing to work as any first responder was trained to do. Actually I don't think it's training at all. I believe it's something within you—a desire to serve discovered way before you enlist. The various organizations just train you to do it well! Tragically, officer Dean, understandably wanting to get to his regular assignment that morning, did not see the collapsed roadway ahead of him. It was just too dark. He drove off the end of the remaining roadway to his death. This interchange is now known as the Clarence Wayne Dean Memorial Interchange. The section of the I-5 collapse left a big rig and several cars stranded on an island of freeway between the downed sections! They later had to be lifted off the 'island' and onto the ground with heavy-duty cranes.

That morning it was one shocking discovery after another. Apparently all the mountaintop microwaves, transmitters, repeater sites got jumbled up as well as everything else. One time I was standing by waiting to go and lost contact with the news room, only to find myself talking to the late, great Charlie Tuna, a local radio icon, on his station's 2- way. I described what I was looking at and then after a minute or two found myself back with KFWB. It was getting a bit crazy! We kept moving around that first hour or two. We saw the collapse of a section of the 118 freeway, more fires, and a multi-story parking lot that had collapsed on itself. We saw emergency lights from fire, police and other first responders zigzagging all over the valley floor.

Every so often Kevin flew over our hangars at the airport to see if any of the other pilots have arrived. Finally we saw that one had. We landed and Kevin hopped out to get the CBS network TV ship going. A pilot who would become a great friend, Glen Galbraith climbed aboard to replace Kevin. After a fresh load of fuel we were off again.

Once back in the air and reporting I got to experience something only those who fly could really appreciate. We had many aftershocks that day and for days after but I'll never forget that first one. I was over a huge and deadly apartment building collapse.

While I was describing what I was seeing, which was a massive search and rescue response by Los Angeles City Fire, the anchor inside the KFWB studio shouted, "Oh. Oh! We're having another one right now! The whole studio is rocking!"

In the helicopter of course we felt nothing but as I looked toward the horizon all of the hills surrounding the San Fernando Valley had walls of dust rising from their bases. It looked like some giant had picked them up and then dropped them to the ground again. Dust and dirt flew everywhere!! Truly amazing!

I saw that same thing happen countless times over the next few days. I saw and tried to describe from "Jet Copter 98" many tragic events that day and during the days that followed. Every corner of life in Los Angeles was impacted in one way or another and was for the many years to follow. LAX, Los Angeles International Airport, one of the busiest Airports in the World had to shut down for a while right after the earthquake. Burbank Airport suffered damage as well. After a few days KFWB got back onto a somewhat normal schedule or 'Clock' in radio speak.

For quite some time after the earthquake my work day began in Jet Copter 98 at 4:00 AM instead of the normal 6:00 AM mostly to try and help the thousands and thousands of drivers coming out of Palmdale, Lancaster and other areas to the north. You have to remember, with sections of the I-5 and the 14 collapsed leading to the merge that got you into the San Fernando Valley only ONE lane of traffic could get through! At 4:00 AM I was astonished to see miles and miles of already stopped motorists inching their way towards what was just a normally busy interchange, with precious few alternatives. The Metrolink rail service was one option and for many the only option. Metro started leasing equipment from Amtrak, Canada and San Francisco to try and keep up with the demand. Rail service to Ventura and Oxnard in place today is a direct result of the Northridge Earthquake and commuter demand. The impact on infrastructure was obvious for all to see but it was the disruption to personal life and way of life that I found extraordinary for years to come.

Marriages came apart, jobs were lost, the simple and basic act of getting up to that alarm buzzer that started this whole story seemed to be just too much for many, many people. A vast understatement but lives were turned upside down. Those that could get to work spent ridiculous amounts of hours just going back and forth. Some took apartments or rented rooms and returned home on weekends only. It really took incredible amounts of faith, trust, love and strength— not muscle strength—but a strength that comes from the heart to get through this, survive and grow.

For me I had it pretty easy. I did get back to my place about two days later. A few of my friends and neighbors had taken the time to go into my apartment and sweep all the broken stuff into large piles that I could go through. They unplugged appliances, taped windows, got the door to almost lock, an unending amount of work. But I did have a home. Oh, remember that image that I thought I saw darting across the living room during the quake? It turned out to be the steel propeller from a 172 Cessna that the mechanics at Jet Copters had painted and signed for me many years before. It weighs about a hundred pounds and yet it danced about 50 feet from hall to front door.

I was emotionally spent just looking at it all. Nancy, I will love you forever for doing so much clean up and repair work before I finally got home. This is a true pitch in and help friend. If we get two or three friends like that going through life we are blessed. I don't know how single parents or grandparents living alone, mobility challenged men, women, and children, pets got through any of this. The list of people who did get through it is endless. This certainly was not the worst tragedy on the world stage but it hit people really hard. I think the ability to look at something that at first blush might seem impossible to overcome and then slowly find a way around, through or live with it for a while, is the most important part of our makeup.

Many, many people did just that in Los Angeles. Lessons were learned, first responders reaped volumes of new information on Search and Rescue. For those of us who did get through all this, I'd say we were better, more prepared for the next roadblock in life. Unfortunately for Los Angeles commuters, though, the 405 is still an ordeal.

 ON THE GROUND WITH MARY!

Any traumatic event produces a ripple effect of reactions. Those of us who experienced the Northridge Earthquake shared to various degrees similar experiences. A couple of glasses in my home broke even though I thought my entire house was coming down. Jeff's home was a minefield of broken glass and in places his building did come down. Other homes were completely destroyed. Our immediate and prolonged reactions to that magnitude 6.7 event were, however, uniquely our own. Some area residents rode it out, picked up whatever had fallen down, and went about their days suffering no problematic reactions. Others experienced mild emotional and cognitive reactions to the event while others continue to suffer from the impact of that event.

The impact of that earthquake wasn't limited to those of us living in the immediate area. Travel to and from Los Angeles was impacted. Businesses suffered. Family life was disrupted. The ripples just kept widening. That's the way it is when just about any event takes place. Everything changes and the ripples just keep going.

One ripple effect was our reactions to the aftershocks. Some of us became really upset. Some of us shrugged them off. Some of us ran for cover. For many of us, our aftershock reactions didn't stop when the aftershocks stopped. A passing truck, a car backfire, a book falling off of a shelf—any one of those everyday events could trigger the fear reactions associated with the original quake. For many people, those trigger events lasted for years after the actual earthquake.

Earlier we talked about our fight or flight reactions to perceived dangers. One of the reasons we startled or even jumped for safety when large trucks rattled our windows was because we remembered the sounds and the physical sensations experienced during that terrifying time. To us that very vivid memory seemed real because of the way the truck sounded. In our minds we were back in the earthquake again. We experienced fear not because passing trucks or falling books or vehicle backfires are inherently dangerous but because our thoughts, based on that previous and frightening event, told us that we were having another earthquake or even that we were having the same earthquake and were in danger.

Such strong fear reactions to situations that present no danger are—put in the most basic terms—all in our heads. Based on previous experiences we interpret current events as dangerous. Once we decide that we're in danger we react accordingly. We can also learn to quickly assess the situation and decide that we are not in danger.

My clinical orientation as a licensed social worker is Cognitive Behavior Therapy. I believe that to a large extent we live life in our heads. We constantly interpret data (events) in order to make sense out of them. All too often our interpretations are skewed by our beliefs, memories, hopes, disappointments, and possibly even by our genetic inheritances. Our thoughts become distorted and therefore our behavior can also lose a certain coherency. That doesn't mean that we are running around living out of control lives because of our thoughts but it might indicate that sometimes our lives become a bit more and unnecessarily complicated because of the way we interpret events—because of the thoughts we use for those interpretations.

All of us on occasion have automatic thoughts. We sometimes rely on rules, assumptions, or beliefs. Most of the time we have no idea we're doing this or even where these thoughts or rules or assumptions or beliefs originated. Most of the time these thoughts don't get in our way. They don't complicate our lives. Sometimes, though, they do. They can seem valid and true and can be associated with uncomfortable feelings and even problematic behaviors. Here are some examples.

Even though we understand that people can't really read our minds, we do on occasion believe we can read the minds of others. Have you ever just decided that you knew what someone was thinking? A friend invites you out for a cup of coffee. You doubt the sincerity of the invitation and immediately conclude that the friend feels sorry for you and is trying to lift your spirits. Come time for the coffee you might even be resentful because you've decided the true motives behind the invitation.

Not too long ago my kitchen sink backed up. The drain appeared to be blocked. I called the plumber and immediately convinced myself the blocked drain was a major problem, which would cost me thousands of dollars. I was utilizing a distorted thought process called catastrophic thinking. I got myself all worked up over the expense. I also decided that all the drains in the house would soon stop working. The problem turned out to be minor and the plumber didn't even charge me. The only expense incurred was the wear and tear on me because of my distorted thinking.

We also believe we must be perfect and loved by everyone. We predict the future and then react as though our predictions were correct. In addition to my catastrophic thoughts about my sink drain, I was also predicting the future by deciding that the plumbing charges would be more than I could afford.

We also personalize events. It was my fault the drain was plugged up. That seems to be easier than acknowledging that I had no idea what happened. I live in an old house. Plumbing problems are not unknown in old houses. However, my first reaction might have been to personalize the problem and blame myself.

We also create rules about how people should behave. Obviously some rules are necessary and helpful. However, it's important to think about why we are doing things and whether or not the things we are doing are helpful.

We can do this by challenging some of our thoughts and beliefs. Learning to restructure distorted thoughts and challenging core beliefs can often help us manage our feelings of anger or depression.

The first step in challenging our thoughts and beliefs is to pay attention to our self-talk. This doesn't necessarily mean that we should talk out loud and pay attention to what we're saying. Self-talk refers to our silent, internal dialogue that goes along with our thoughts. Generally our self-talk is in words. Pay attention to the words you use as you talk yourself through the day. Do you criticize yourself or praise yourself? Is your self-talk giving you more confidence or is it undermining your sense of self? At first, just notice the words used for your self-talk.

Next try identifying some habitual thought patterns. These are the thoughts that seem almost automatic. For example, if you head out the door without your keys do you tell yourself that you always do stupid things or do you simply without blame just go back and get them. If your habitual thought is that you are stupid and do stupid things you aren't going to feel particularly good about yourself. We wouldn't like it if another person kept putting us down and yet we often say things that put ourselves down.

We think ourselves through the day and we talk ourselves through the day. Our thoughts have a direct impact on our feelings and on our behaviors. We interpret events with thoughts. Our thoughts lead to feelings and behaviors, which can create an entirely new event to which we have thoughts which lead to feelings and so goes our days.

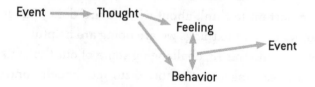

We know all too well that we can't control the majority of events in our lives. Drivers run red lights. People we love become ill and die. Jobs come and go. The alarm clock doesn't go off. The coffee maker stops working. Significant things happen. Insignificant things happen. We have thoughts about all of them. While we can't change many of the events of our lives, we can change the way we think about those events.

We don't have to feel so angry that we throw a lamp. We don't have to feel so helpless that we give up. We don't have to feel that our lives lack meaning. Those feelings come from our thoughts about events or they come from beliefs we've held for years. We can change all of that. Such change takes time and patience and practice but it is possible.

Let's start right now by looking at some irrational beliefs we may use to get us through the day. Check off any that seem familiar.

- I've got to be completely competent or perfect in what I do.
- I need to be loved and accepted by others.
- It's easier to avoid problems than to deal with them directly.
- If someone is unhappy it's my fault.
- Life isn't good if I can't quickly solve my problems.
- If something bad happened in the past it will probably happen again.

Checking even one of those beliefs doesn't mean you're a bad person or stupid or weird. It just means that you're human. It also suggests that you might want to challenge those beliefs because they aren't particularly helpful. You can learn to look at events objectively by recognizing your automatic thoughts.

There are countless ways of restructuring unrealistic or distorted thoughts and beliefs. The main thing to remember is that if we can become more aware of our thought patterns, of the words we use in those thought patterns and of our core beliefs we might find that getting through the day can become a little easier.

Once in awhile the ground shakes because of an earthquake. Most of the time, though, a truck is just going past our building. We can decide how we think about the events of our lives. We can make the glorious journey a little easier and we can be kinder to ourselves.

THE STATION FIRE ≫≫

LISTEN UP! HERE IT IS!

California is no stranger to brush fires. Every year plants die and then sprout again creating a buildup of dead vegetation. Many of those plants participating in this cycle are not indigenous to the state and thus disrupt the normal cycle of growth, death, and regrowth. Periodic fires are natural and many plants native to the state depend upon fire to reproduce. Research indicates, however, that these non-native plants have significantly altered the intensity and frequency of the state's wildfires.

Every year homes are threatened if not destroyed. However, the year 2009 was particularly horrible. From early February until late November a series of 8,291 wildfires burned more than 632 square miles and caused an estimated 135 million dollars in damage. Hundreds of structures were destroyed. More than 130 people were injured and 2 people died.

California is the third largest state in the country. It is over 800 miles in length. Those 2009 fires were scattered over the entire area. Although the fires burned in many different regions of the state, August was especially notable for several very large fires in Southern California.

In Southern California, the normal wildfire season begins in October with the arrival of the infamous Santa Ana winds. It's unusual for fires to get out of control at other times of the year. However, during the 2009 firestorms temperatures throughout the southern part of the state were above 100 degrees for much of August. These high temperatures combined with low humidity and large amounts of dead vegetation, some of which had not burned for decades, created a perfect environment for normal fires to quickly explode out of control even without winds to spread the flames. These conditions combined with the rugged terrain of many areas made firefighting extremely difficult.

The Station Fire in the Los Angeles area was the largest and deadliest of those wildfires. It began in the Angeles National Forest near a ranger station above La Canada Flintridge on August 26. That particular area had not experienced a major fire in more than sixty years. In a matter of hours it grew to more than 100,000 acres. It wasn't declared 'out' until October 16. During that time it burned 251 square miles. Two firefighters (Captain Tedmund Hall and Firefighter Specialist Arnie Quinones) lost their lives battling the blaze.

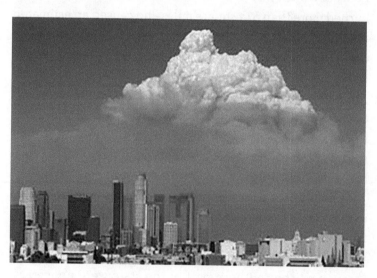

Plumes of thick smoke spiraled at least 20,000 feet in the air. In fact, the smoke from the Station Fire was visible to and photographed by NASA's Terra satellite 438 miles above the Earth's surface. In addition to forcing thousands of evacuations and threatening thousands of homes and buildings, the fire also threatened to burn the major communications installations on Mount Wilson. Had the Mount Wilson towers burned and collapsed, much of the Los Angeles basin would have become silent. Mount Wilson is home to 20 television and radio transmission towers and a vast assortment of fire and police communications equipment. It is also home to the Mount Wilson Observatory.

Mike Dietrich, the U.S. Forest Service Incident Commander, described the fire as angry and said that, "Until we get a change in weather conditions, I'm not overly optimistic. The fire pretty much goes wherever it wants. It's like it has a mind of its own."

As the hot weather continued, it seemed that the only atmospheric changes were those created by the fire itself. The Station Fire created its own wind patterns. The determined cause of this most devastating of fires is that it was man made. It ranks as the largest fire in Los Angeles County history. In addition to the two lives lost, it destroyed over two dozen homes, burned an area nearly the size of Chicago, and cut off access to one of the most popular wilderness gateways in the Los Angeles area. The fire was so hot that it not only destroyed trees but also the tree roots. Indeed, the Station Fire changed forever the landscape of Los Angeles County.

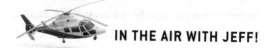

IN THE AIR WITH JEFF!

Fires are terrifying to report on. From the air they become surreal. You are out of harm's way, high above in a helicopter or airplane trying to convey to the listener that they just might be in harm's way! Reporting on fires is extremely dynamic. Something is always moving beneath you: Flame, smoke, wind, people, animals and first responders. If the fire starts out as a brush fire and then continues to destroy homes and life, the event becomes extraordinary. It touches those directly involved and in a different way those simply observing the tragedy. When a home is destroyed by fire, it's more than wood, plaster and building materials. You're watching someone's life just disappearing before your eyes. A note from your dad, a picture of Grandma, a memento of your life . . . countless objects that you could always turn to . . . now gone. Having covered so many different types of fires over the last 20 plus years in Los Angeles and surrounding counties, a few really stand out. They make you grateful for the bed you climb into at night and that picture of mom standing next to the airplane she soloed in many years ago!

A fire that hit a section of Malibu, California one windy night is one that is always with me. As usual in this part of Los Angeles County, when the Santa Ana winds start to blow, sometimes with gusts to over 50 MPH, they enter the San Fernando Valley in the northeast corner near Sylmar and the Newhall Pass, travel southwest across the west San Fernando Valley and finally out to the Pacific Ocean and Malibu. Along the way they get squeezed thru passes and canyons, up slopes and down slopes getting super charged by the topography along the way. The flames feed on usually dry brush. By the time the wind driven fire hits the Santa Monica Mountains, the news station term "out of control wild fire" is an understatement!

This night what started out as what should have been a rather innocent vehicle fire, alongside Pacific Coast Highway near The Bluffs Park, went from a routine call to the Fire Department to destroying several homes and damaging several more in just an hour or so. Luckily for the rest of Malibu and the people that live there, the fire went down slope towards Malibu road, over it in a flash and onto the small strip of beach front homes and finally into the Pacific Ocean. The fire received a lot of media coverage including some national coverage due mostly to its incredible speed and the fame of a few of the homeowners directly involved.

Weeks could go by and then a funk would come over me that I would learn was a bit of depression thinking of those that lost the notes, pictures and mementos in a few hours of a windy night. The other side of that experience was the largest brush fire in Los Angeles County fire history—The Station Fire.

There has been and still is a vicious cycle of weather in Los Angeles believe it or not. It is warm and dry most of the year but during what is the fall for most of our country, strange things begin to happen in Southern California. First the wind starts to blow, followed by the wind blowing hard, followed by the dreaded Santa Ana winds. The howl generally speaking comes from the Northeast to the Southwest. Writers with skill much greater than mine have described them in fiction and fact but trust me, they just make the average Jane and Joe feel weird and 'on edge' a tad. So first it's wind, followed by great fires, some reaching historic numbers then later or near the top of the New Year comes the rain. The rain never seems to come in nice, sensible showers but it arrives in great intense storms that overpower the areas that really need the water and have yet to figure out how to save it or store it. Most of it winds up in Long Beach harbor!

Reporting these great rains, floods, mud slides, landslides, home slides and unending chaos keeps Los Angeles newsrooms churning out things like "Team coverage, Storm Watch 2014!" Traffic in and around Los Angeles is the NUMBER ONE social issue! From school age children to parents, professionals to City, County, State workers and elected officials and yes even Jennifer Anniston trying to get to the studio, the first question is . . . "What's the traffic like and where do I park??" When these weather events hit, all bets are off.

Earlier in this section we described the enormity of the Station Fire. There's a kind of ennui in the early stages of a fire. We've been there so many times before that we assume we know what will happen next in those early stages. By day two, however, I was confronted with the unthinkable—a massive out of control wild fire starting to ramp up big time.

Late in the afternoon on that August day in 2009 I spotted some smoke up in the Angeles National Forest as we were taking off for the afternoon shift. Our newsroom was getting some calls from people who could see the smoke as well. Indications were that some brush was burning alongside Angeles Crest Highway above La Canada Flintridge. As it turned out the origin was close to a Ranger Station in the mountains. That point of origin gave it the name—The Station Fire.

As we flew above it I reported on what I could see. It was quite active. There was a lot of flame, smoke and fuel (dry brush) but the all-important wind was nowhere near a Santa

Ana condition! Windy, yes, but manageable. I thought the responding fire attack would be able to get a handle on it before nightfall. The "handle on it" didn't come for the better part of a month after burning 251 square miles (160,000 acres), burning 89 homes and 209 other structures, and killing 2 firefighters as they tried to retreat from advancing flames by driving off a narrow mountain road covered in smoke and flame. Roads were closed for more than a year and a long investigation would follow all the fire jurisdictions involved.

The fire was extremely tough for the media to cover, describe and photograph due to the fact that the station fire for the most part was a fuel driven fire rather than one pushed and directed by high winds. The incredible amount of smoke just rose directly over the fire obscuring what was burning. In the end the Station Fire was the 10th largest Wildfire in modern Los Angeles history. The next year parts of La Canada Flintridge, Tujunga and Glendale were inundated with mudslides pouring off the now naked hillside where trees and brush had once held it all together. In Los Angeles one must be extremely careful where one builds and lives.

A mudslide is an almost silent monster that slowly gathers everything in its path downhill until it arrives at the rear of your home and then proceeds to go right through it taking lives and home along with it.

I went home after a day of fire reporting, got into my bed and started thinking: "Gosh, there are people out there who don't have this anymore. People who have lost everything they had, everything they have ever worked for."

That's what really brings it home for me.

There was one cul-de-sac in Altadena hit by the firestorm. As soon as it broke we flew over the zone. I looked down and saw 15 homes burned down to their slab foundations. But one home was intact and the owner was standing outside with a small child.

As we went over, he looked up at us, put out his arms and shrugged like he couldn't believe it himself.

Every moment we were seeing people of great courage. In every fire people who had been asked to evacuate their homes just chose to stay with their property and remained up there with their hoses and buckets of water. That's someone taking a stand and saying: "Wait a minute, this is mine and I want to protect it and I'm going to keep it." That, to me, is amazing. Unfortunately, if the situation gets bad fast such decisions can put the first responders at great risk if they have to go back in and rescue those who refused to evacuate.

I was also impressed and confused by the relentless nature of the fire. I remember a moment during the Station Fire when the flames climbed back into the San Gabriel Mountains and marched right up them while the wind was blowing down the mountains in complete contradiction. You can never figure it. It made no sense.

But now that it's all over, my personal relief comes from knowing there's an end to the anxiety and the human suffering.

 ON THE GROUND WITH MARY!

For decades I lived in an extreme fire hazard area of Los Angeles County. After sixty homes in my neighborhood were destroyed in a wildfire I was unable to obtain fire insurance without going through the State of California's insurance program. Packing up to evacuate became a bizarre routine for my family and me. The first time we readied to evacuate we determined that an astonishing number of possessions were essential. The car was loaded with keepsakes and documents and computers as well as pets. We were good to go. The next time we repeated the drill we couldn't help but notice that the essentials had become fewer until, finally, we got the pets ready to travel and that was it.

This change of what was essential happened because there's only so much stuff you can lug around. I went to my bank and rented a safety deposit box for all of the essential papers. I replaced my desk computer with a laptop and then I ultimately I didn't even bother with the laptop because I'd obtained a remote backup for a very small annual fee. I scanned irreplaceable photographs, which were then backed up by my remote service.

These changes reduced the number of irreplaceable items to those living in the house. That made getting ready to evacuate much easier. It also made daily living much easier because I no longer had to worry about my possessions. Of course, I still have a lot of 'stuff' but knowing that none of it really matters that much is very liberating. Friends and family are often confounded or amused by the number of books in my library but the books are certainly not rare, first editions. They can be replaced. Or I can check them out of a public library. What matters are the living beings inside the house.

Years of getting ready to evacuate and on a few occasions actually evacuating taught me that lesson. I now know the things I value. I also now know more about my entire value system. I think that by taking a good, hard look at the possessions we value we might have an opportunity—without a wildfire—of discovering more about what we value in life. I believe that our values determine the actions we take, as well as the goals we set. Values vary from person to person and even from community to community and country to country.

Here are some exercises you might like to try. As always, there's no pressure. We're not looking over your shoulder. If they don't appeal to you, just skip them and read on.

List three valuables that you would want to take with you if your home suddenly caught on fire.

1. ....

2. ....

3. ....

Let's move from valuables (meaning possessions) to values. By values I mean principles or ethics. List three values that you believe to be typically American. There is no right or wrong answer to this. It's just your opinion.

1. ....

2. ....

3. ....

Now think back to your teenage years. List two values you had as a teenager but which no longer seem that important to you.

1. ....

2. ....

Now list three values that you think are or were important to your parents.

1. ....

2. ....

3. ....

And finally list your five current most important values.

1. ....

2. ....

3. ....

4. ....

5. ....

If you created these lists you might have noticed that there's a difference between our valuables and our values and that both are fluid. The valuables I held dear when I was a child are not that important to me now. If they were still around I probably wouldn't take them with me if I had to evacuate.

My values (those standards by which I try to live) also tend to change throughout the years. During adolescence peer approval might have been high on my list of values. Today living with integrity might be higher up on the list. Also chances are some of the values held by my parents no longer to apply. For example, my parents may have not have placed self-care high on their list of values. Their generation wasn't well known for its high level of self-care. For me, taking good care of my physical, mental and emotional health is important. That level of self-care enables me to be present for the people I love. Honesty was definitely high on my parents' value list and it remains high on mine.

The possessions we value as well as the standards or ethics we value do change, though, with time. Even with that somewhat fluid nature, I believe that we are in some way defined by both the possessions we value as well as by our ethics—our values.

Here's a list of values. Take a look at it. Some of them might be important to you. Others might not seem that significant.

Wisdom	Wealth	Being Trustworthy
Skill	Religious Faith	Recognition
Power	Pleasure	Physical Appearance
Morality	Loyalty	Love
Knowledge	Justice	Honesty
Health	Creativity	Job
Family	Education	Achievement

We've left you some room to write in some values not on the list. This list might help you if you want to write down your most important values. Remember that years from now the list might change. Job and achievement might be high on the list today and in several years family and health might top the list. It's your list. We're not keeping score.

However, since this book is all about change I think it's important to know who you are and to know what's important to you. Change, as we've discovered, is hard. Knowing what's important to you can make the changes you choose to make so much easier. And you won't ever have to run back into a burning building to rescue your values because they are always with you.

THE O. J. SLOW CHASE

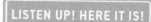

On June 13, 1994, shortly after midnight, the blood-soaked bodies of Nicole Brown Simpson (former wife of football great O. J. Simpson) and Ronald Goldman were discovered in the exclusive Brentwood area of Los Angeles. They had both been stabbed to death on the Spanish-tile walkway leading to Nicole Brown Simpson's Bundy Drive home while her two children slept in their rooms.

Police tried to contact O. J. Simpson only to discover he had left for Chicago on a flight leaving a little before midnight that same night. Forensic evidence indicated that Brown and Goldman had died around ten o'clock that evening. Law enforcement was able to contact Simpson to tell him of his ex-wife's death. He returned to Los Angeles a little before noon the following day. When he arrived at his home he was taken into police custody for questioning. He was later released.

Shortly after his release, Simpson hired attorney Robert Shapiro. As the police continued their investigation evidence began to point to O. J. as a suspect: Bloodstains on the walkway where the bodies were found matched Simpson's. Two bloodstained gloves were recovered—one at the scene and the other outside Simpson's Brentwood home. Drops of blood on his driveway and inside his home matched Nicole Brown Simpson's blood type.

As police gathered more evidence pointing toward him, O. J. started treatment for depression. Four days after the bodies were discovered, he attended his ex-wife's funeral. Later he appeared to go into a depression so deep that his attorney sent several doctors to the friend's home where Simpson had been staying. The friend was Robert Kardashian. O. J. appeared to be heavily sedated and remained at the Kardashian home. A short time later Los Angeles police officers wrapped up their investigation with the recommendation that O. J. Simpson be charged with two counts of first-degree murder.

On Friday, June 17, 1994, at 8:30 AM, Los Angeles Police authorities informed Robert Shapiro that O. J. Simpson must surrender by 11:00 that morning. Arraignment was scheduled in Los Angeles Municipal Court that afternoon. Shapiro immediately went to Kardashian's home where O. J. was just waking up. He informed O. J. that he must turn himself in at Parker Center. An hour went by during which O. J. talked on the phone to his children, his mother, and his personal attorney. He made changes to his will. He wrote several letters.

As the eleven o'clock deadline approached, thousands of reporters gathered at Parker Center. When Shapiro received a phone call from the Los Angeles Police Department asking about Simpson's whereabouts he replied that doctors were examining him. Police arrived a few minutes later to take O. J. into custody. Shapiro, Kardashian and Simpson's friend Al Cowlings were told that they could accompany Simpson to Parker Center. Cowlings, a former teammate at the University of Southern California as well as the Buffalo Bills, went into another room to bring Simpson out. After several minutes a psychiatrist went into the room to assist Cowlings. Neither O. J. nor Cowlings was in the room. They had apparently left the house through a back door and driven off in a white Ford Bronco.

Robert Shapiro immediately arranged a press conference to announce that he feared Simpson might commit suicide.

During the press conference, Kardashian read a handwritten note Simpson had left behind.

> "I think of my life and feel I've done most of the right things. So why do I end up like this? I can't go on. No matter what the outcome, people will look and point. I can't take that. I can't subject my children to that. I have nothing to do with the murder. I love her. Don't feel sorry for me. I've had a great life. Please think of the real O. J. and not this lost person. Thanks for making my life special. I hope I helped yours. Peace and love, O. J."

Early that afternoon Los Angeles Police spokesman, Commander David Gascon, issued an all points bulletin and announced that O. J. Simpson was officially a fugitive wanted on suspicion of murder.

Several hours later an Orange County motorist reported seeing Simpson as a passenger in a white Ford Bronco. The motorist believed the Bronco was driven by Al Cowlings. A few minutes later a police officer saw the Bronco going north on the 405 freeway. He approached the vehicle with sirens and lights. Cowlings yelled out the window that Simpson was in the back seat of the vehicle holding a gun to his own head. The officer backed off to follow the Bronco.

Thus began one of the strangest car chases in the history of Los Angeles car chases. Eventually at least 20 police cars, never going more than 35 miles an hour, followed the Bronco. Every moment of the chase was televised and throughout the country people sat mesmerized in front of their television sets. Bars and stores and shopping malls filled with people just watching the chase. Not wanting to miss even one minute of the chase coverage, television viewers ordered dinner delivered. One pizza delivery chain reported deliveries equal to Super Bowl Sunday. Life seemed to stop. Traffic definitely stopped. The Southern California skies filled with news and law enforcement aircraft. Spectators crowded onto freeway overpasses hoping to catch a glimpse of the white Ford Bronco and its flashing light entourage.

Late that evening Cowlings, still followed by law enforcement and media, pulled into the cobblestone driveway of Simpson's mansion. Law enforcement surrounded the vehicle and watched while Cowlings got out and walked into the house. Simpson, pistol in hand, stayed in the Bronco for almost an hour. A little before 9:00 PM Los Angeles Police Department Special Weapons and Tactics team and negotiators persuaded Simpson to put down his gun and get out of the Bronco. When he did leave the vehicle the only thing in his hands was a framed family photograph.

Police allowed Simpson to go into his house to use the bathroom, call his mother, and drink a glass of orange juice. After an hour inside his home, he was transported to Parker Center and booked on two counts of murder.

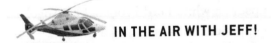 ## IN THE AIR WITH JEFF!

We all have been watching police chase bad guys for years and years. Mack Sennett put it all to film after the turn of the century and the rest is history. It proved to be entertainment of the highest order. Car chases are sometimes amusing and, at least for me, always amazing. They appear dangerous and the outcome is always doubtful.

In 1999 one of my favorite television shows was a situation comedy called "It's Like, You Know". It only lasted one season and I loved it! The pretty vacuous story line involved life in Los Angeles seen through the eyes of a diehard New Yorker. One entire episode was about a pursuit. Every single scene had the pursuit playing on a television in the background and every single person's reaction to it played out. Whether the scenes took place in bars, schools, courtrooms, or hospital operating rooms everyone was engrossed in the pursuit. Some of the characters knew the police lingo and were explaining to others what would happen next.

I think that episode came close to accurately reflecting how we in Southern California feel about car chases. Whether we're watching them on television or from freeway overpasses or listening to them on radio, we can't turn away. We are captivated by the car chase. Perhaps we can all either thank or blame poor old Mack Sennett for this collective fascination with pursuit.

The pursuit I'm about to try and do justice to had the attention of all the major United States television networks, most local television outlets, some foreign television networks, countless radio outlets, and over 100 million viewers and listeners around the world. The center of all this attention was O. J. Simpson, a white Ford Bronco, Los Angeles freeways and a lot of police!! It was the O. J. Pursuit.

Early in the morning of June 13, 1994, I was beginning my shift with KFWB News 98. As you'll remember from some of these earlier stories the first thing for me to do was get all my radios and scanners going and check in with the news desk to see if there were any assignments for me. There had already been a police item on most newsroom's desks about a rather gruesome sounding murder in the trendy community of Brentwood. What got the attention of most assignment desks was one of those killed was the former wife of one

Orenthal James Simpson or as he was better known on this planet "O. J." There was another victim at the time described as an adult male. I was given the address and asked the pilot to go as directly as possible towards Brentwood from Van Nuys. We were on scene in about 4 minutes. My first responsibility is to provide the station with a "sitrep" and advise the editor if indeed there is something going on and at what level. From there I can cover it until reporters arrive on the ground and the story plays out.

My first chat with the newsroom went something like this, "It's a quiet street in Brentwood, just off South Bundy Drive and Montana Avenue, near the eastern side of Brentwood Country Club. There's a crime scene set up around the address and a lot of LAPD black and whites but the unusual part is the number of unmarked detective/supervisor cars. There is a lot going on here!!"

For years, this story would play and play and play. There was of course an intensive investigation well under way. The crime had been committed in the early morning hours. Our newsroom knew most of this already but hearing it from my vantage point and from the vantage points of some local TV ships now transmitting pictures made this THE story with all hands on deck.

It wasn't too long before the victims were identified as Nicole Brown Simpson, ex-wife of O. J. and Ronald Goldman, who was initially identified as a waiter at a nearby Brentwood restaurant. For the next four or five days the story played out with LAPD detectives relaying information as they could but one unusual aspect started getting bigger and bigger. O. J. Simpson himself was being questioned and slowly but surely becoming a suspect! O. J. Simpson a suspect? It was getting a bit hard to follow but it really ramped up when on June 17 O. J. was supposed to turn himself in to LAPD headquarters and failed to appear.

Up to this point my job was just to keep tabs on the home of Nicole Brown Simpson, the crime scene and Simpson's home for any signs of abnormal behavior. Nothing really happened. However, when O. J. failed to appear and became a fugitive every newsroom in the country lit up.

KFWB editors and news directors said to me, "Let's find him!"

The search was on!! We knew all the locations of the major players involved in the story—the lawyers, the friends, and the family. We flew all afternoon hoping to come up with something. Every now and then the newsroom would call me on the 2 way and say that a caller had spotted O. J. here or there. The locations were from all corners of Los Angeles County.

At one point I remember one editor saying, "It's getting like Elvis sightings. It's insane!"

Well a little after six that afternoon, someone did spot that white Bronco with two men inside and one was O. J. Simpson. They were traveling north now from southern Orange County and CHP had confirmed all this.

The first hint I heard on scanner channels was, "We got him. We're right behind. Driver says O. J. has a gun."

The next five plus hours crept by for me. At that time KFWB ran two airborne units. My pilot and I were in a Bell Jet Ranger 206 B-3 and Lisa Walker and her pilot were in a 172 Cessna. Lisa was based out of Fullerton Airport and I out of Van Nuys Airport. When I heard that hit on the scanner and called our newsroom we were on short final to Van Nuys Airport for fuel and Lisa was about to wrap the afternoon shift at Fullerton. The newsroom and I were instantly calling Lisa asking her to not land but to pick up the pursuit because she was close by.

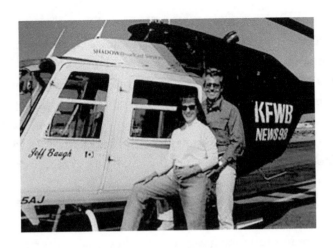

In our excitement we were stepping all over each other on the same frequency. Lisa's pilot was on short final to Fullerton Airport and actually waved the landing while over the threshold to continue flying with the bit of fuel they had left. Lisa was over the pursuit while we refueled at Van Nuys Airport. The plan was for Lisa to cover the Bronco until they had just enough fuel to get back to Fullerton without incident. Then we would pick it up from there with full fuel tanks. At this point we're sitting at Van Nuys Airport in a running helicopter. (Hot fueling was allowed then.) I'm listening to Lisa, to the desk and to a scanner that has exploded with voice on this incident and I'm watching and hearing Wayne Richardson, the pilot, screaming at the poor pump guy to make the fuel go in the tanks faster! Wow! What a scene! The world now knew what was happening in Los Angeles. Every TV station and every radio station was all over this. NBC was in the middle of broadcasting game #5 of the NBA Finals between the Knicks and the Rockets and switched to a SPLIT SCREEN! Tom Brokaw, doing the evening news, got the big section of the picture and the playoff game got the small box! (Note: Just to illustrate what television executives think about the strength of a pursuit on ratings, years after the O. J. chase President George W. Bush was giving one of his most important announcements on stem cell research while we were covering a pursuit that went from Los Angeles into Ventura County before the driver surrendered. The television networks switched to split screen and the President got the small box so Southern California viewers wouldn't miss the car chase!!)

Meanwhile back at the O. J. chase. Lisa Walker in Air 98 was and continues to be my hero. Lisa later retired and took on a much tougher assignment a few years after this all played out. She became a full-time mom to two beautiful children!

So now we go back to the Bronco! Lisa is now almost over the pursuit coming north from Orange County, using the 5, the 405 and now the west bound 91. She is live on KFWB describing the scene, which has turned from pursuit as we know it to more of a slow speed pursuit with a following which soon became a parade of sorts through the rush hours of Los Angeles. The sheer number of people stopping to watch this all go by was astonishing. The spectators clogged and stopped freeway overpasses trying to get near the infamous white Bronco. Lisa continued to describe the freeway procession as it headed toward LAX. The white Bronco was followed closely by a chevron of CHP and police vehicles from many jurisdictions, motor officers, reporters in various vehicles, and a variety of media vans.

At times people just ran onto the freeways shouting encouragement to O. J. Airspace above the cavalcade was as busy as the freeway on which it inched along. Every single news outlet—local and national radio, television, and print—with a helicopter or airplane was represented in that crowded airspace. A lot of private aircraft pilots joined the fray just because they could. All of this is moving through the skies and freeways of Los Angeles in the late afternoon! It seemed that the only thing missing was the Goodyear Blimp! I seriously expected at any moment to see it alongside. All anyone curious about O.J.'s location had to do was look towards the sky over the South Bay at the swarm of aircraft, strobes, and position lights flashing away to know exactly where he was! By now, most of us and perhaps half the country had figured out that O. J. Simpson was headed for his Brentwood home. LAPD was, of course, way ahead of us. We would all later learn about its running dialog with O. J. and his family members. The KFWB desk had sent reporters to his home to be on scene when he did arrive. So did all other Los Angeles media!

Lisa has now pulled off the event just south of LAX and landed safely at Fullerton Airport completely out of breath and fuel. We picked up the event now coming towards LAX on the northbound 405 and the LAX air traffic controllers, who knew we were coming, graciously cleared us all through to the north as one gigantic flight of aircraft! With these words we had become one, gigantic multi-craft flying machine: "LAX, this is a media flight of 23 or 24, we'd like to transition north through your airspace and clear to Santa Monica!"

The 405 was still clogged with drivers pulling off to the shoulders to get a glimpse of the spectacle. It must be noted that 'tweeting' and all other forms of social media had not yet taken over our lives. This was doubtless a gift and helped drivers avoid the horrible accidents that would have happened if all of those 'gawkers' and been taking pictures and 'tweeting' and posting on social media. Let's not forget that my primary job is to help drivers get around or avoid problems. This congested situation was dangerous enough. If it had happened today I think there would have been many more accidents and tragedies. As an aside, my radio listeners are almost always in cars trying to get from one place to another. That's the main reason they are listening to my broadcasts. Television viewers aren't behind the wheel and are presumably safe.

I often feel torn between keeping my listeners out of trouble and accurately describing events. This slow chase on increasingly crowded freeways and streets was no exception. And the crowds were still building. Everything was getting harder to contain or manage and we're still north on the 405 headed to the Sunset Boulevard off ramp. This enormous procession is now exiting the North 405 at Sunset. This part has all the ingredients for something bad about to happen. Spectators were all over Sunset Boulevard with LAPD and CHP trying to control this chaotic event trying to prevent someone being hit and injured. There are civilian motorcyclists driving like flies buzzing around food. Some people probably don't know what is going on or even who O. J. Simpson is and they are intermingled with all the other people who are there taking in the sights. Somehow this entire group of cars, motorcycles, police, spectators and people running next to all these vehicles proceeds west bound on Sunset heading towards Simpson's Rockingham home. Finally the white Bronco, driven this entire time by Simpson friend A. C. (Al) Cowlings enters the driveway of O. J.'s home and comes to a stop. A male family member immediately approached the Bronco but was quickly pulled back by LAPD officers who were on the property but not surrounding the vehicle as phone negotiations continued.

While I'm in the air describing what I see all the drama and tension below immediately ramps up. On the ground, KFWB reporter Pete Demetrio is close to the driveway.

He is frantically calling the editor and shouting, "Come to me NOW!"

The anchors shifted to Pete who then announced that O. J. had just surrendered to LAPD without incident. O. J. was under arrest. He was driven to Parker Center LAPD headquarters in downtown Los Angeles. As a reporter, the last I saw of O. J. was when he was led into Men's Central Jail later that evening. His hands cuffed behind him, he disappeared through the doors. The investigation and trial would continue to captivate the world.

 ## ON THE GROUND WITH MARY!

Back in the day when I was young and arrogant, I thought it was pretty funny to stop on a crowded sidewalk and stare into the sky above me or at a building nearby. It never failed. After a few moments passersby would stop and follow my line of sight to see what I saw. Of course, I was looking at nothing in particular. Nevertheless the more people who stood looking the more people joined them. I found this aspect of human behavior fascinating.

There's a similar human behavior involving stopped traffic. The reason for the stop may be as minor as debris in the road or as major as a catastrophic automobile accident. Regardless of the reason, traffic going in the direction opposite from the stopped cars will also grind to a halt. People must get a good look at whatever it is on the other side that caused traffic to stop. We call those opposite direction drivers the 'lookie loos'.

We are all natural voyeurs. We like to see what's going on. Even if we're not interested in the event and even if it's none of our business, we stop. We join the 'lookie loos'. We become part of the 'checking it out' crowd.

Becoming part of a crowd is okay as long as we remember that we are not the crowd—as long as we remember that we can and should think for ourselves. When we forget to think for ourselves or when we allow the group to think for us we can make decisions or exhibit behaviors we may later regret.

In 1972 social psychologist Irving Janis coined the term 'Groupthink'. Groupthink, according to Janis, occurs when members of a group make unwise decisions because of perceived or actual group pressure. Dr. Janis believed that this type of decision-making caused mental inefficiency, faulty reality testing and impaired moral judgment. With Groupthink as its guide members of the group tend to ignore alternatives and engage in behaviors that dehumanize other groups. Going along with the crowd can feel comfortable but can lead us down paths we would not ordinarily travel.

Jerry B. Harvey, PhD. (1935-2015) was Professor Emeritus of Management at The George Washington University. His story of a family car ride from Coleman, Texas, to Abilene, Texas, famously illustrates the difficulty of going against the perceived will of the group. (*The Abilene Paradox and Other Meditations On Management* by Jerry B. Harvey was published by Lexington Books in 1988.) Sometimes it's really hard to not follow the crowd.

Here's my version of Dr. Harvey's family drive to Abilene, Texas.

This summer afternoon in Coleman, Texas, was hot. The thermometer nailed to the outside wall of the drug store read 104 degrees. A hot, dry, wind blew dust through the house and made it feel even hotter. We had a fan going on the back porch and a pitcher of cold lemonade so not only was the afternoon bearable it was at times almost pleasant. We had just about everything we could ask for on this hot, Texas afternoon.

Just about when we had settled in, though, my father-in-law suddenly said, "Let's get in the car and go to Abilene and have dinner at the cafeteria."

I thought, "What, go to Abilene? Fifty-three miles? In this dust storm and heat? And in an unairconditioned 1958 Buick?"

But my wife chimed in with, "Sounds like a great idea. I'd like to go. How about you, Jerry?"

Obviously what I wanted didn't match what the others wanted, so I replied, "Sounds good to me," and kind of desperately added, "I just hope your mother wants to go."

"Of course I want to go," said my mother-in-law. "I haven't been to Abilene in a long time."

So we climbed into the car and headed for Abilene. The heat was brutal. In no time at all we were covered with dust. By the time we got to Abilene our sweat had turned the dust into cement. We struggled into the cafeteria and filled our plates with food that tasted as bad as it looked.

Several hours and many miles later we got back to the house in Coleman. We were hot and dirty and exhausted. For a long time we just sat in front of the fan. It seemed like no one was capable of speech.

Finally the silence got to me and I said, "It was a pretty great trip, wasn't it?"

No one spoke. Everyone just stared at me. Their eyes were red with dust and heat.

Finally, my mother-in-law said, "Well, to tell the truth, I

didn't enjoy it much. I would rather have stayed here. You all seemed to really want to go and I guess I let you pressure me into it. Otherwise I wouldn't have gone."

Stunned, I replied, "What do you mean, you all? I didn't want to go. I only went to please the rest of you."

My wife stared at me in disbelief and finally said, "You were the ones who wanted to go. I just went along to keep you happy. I'm not crazy enough to want to go out in this heat."

Finally my father-in-law slapped the arm of his chair and said, "Hell! I never wanted to go to Abilene. I just thought you might be bored. I wanted to stay here but I guess I wanted to please you all more."

We all sat in silence again. Chances are each one of us was wondering why we had just taken a 106 mile drive across a hot, windy, dusty desert in a car more like a blast furnace than a vehicle to eat terrible food in a place we didn't even want to visit in the first place.

That's my version of Dr. Harvey's Abilene Paradox. No one in that family did what they wanted to do on that hot afternoon. Instead, each family member did what they thought would please the others. The end result was that no one was happy. No one was pleased.

I'm not proposing that the thousands of people lining the streets and freeway overpasses to catch a glimpse or a white Ford Bronco going by or the millions of people glued to their television sets getting even better views of the Bronco creeping along were victims of Groupthink. I will hazard a guess, though, that a great many of those thousands or millions were lining or glued because 'it was the thing to do'. They were embracing their inner voyeur.

Groupthink is the metaphor I gleaned from the O. J. Chase. While group consensus is essential for many decisions, it is equally necessary to remember to think for yourself. Going with the crowd might feel really good. If the crowd is going someplace you don't want to be, though, step aside. That can be really hard sometimes but, seriously, do you really want to wind up someplace you didn't want to be in the first place?

Jeff can attest to how often people just stay stuck in traffic even though there might be multiple opportunities to take a different route and move away from the hazard to arrive safely at the intended destination. I think Groupthink plays a part in that behavior. It seems easier and feels safer to just go along with the group.

Dr. Janis proposed several ways to identify Groupthink: (1) Group members feel overly confident which may lead to its taking dangerous risks. (2) Group members ignore warnings and don't reconsider their beliefs. (3) Group members are so convinced they are right that they ignore the ethical or moral

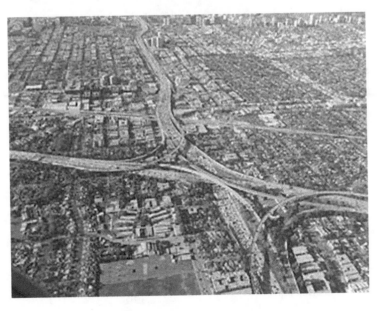

consequences of their decisions. (4) Group members believe that anyone who disagrees with the group is the enemy. (5) Group members feel pressure to not disagree with the group's views. (6) Members of the group protect it.

Groupthink is expedient if the goal is decision and action. In fact, Groupthink is most likely to occur if the group is under pressure to make a decision. Under that type of pressure group members cling all the more tightly to the security of the group.

Think back to a time when you felt insecure or frightened. Were you more or less likely to take a stand? Life can be pretty scary at times and being part of a group can feel like a comfort. The path to comfort, though, isn't always the best road for us to travel.

Watch out. Think for yourself. Be safe.

THE JET BLUE LANDING GEAR »»

JetBlue Airways Flight 292 departed Bob Hope Airport at 3:17 in the afternoon headed for John F. Kennedy International Airport (JFK) in New York City. Aboard the aircraft were 140 passengers and 6 crewmembers. Seconds after take-off, pilot in command, Captain Scott Burke, knew that his Airbus A320-232 was in trouble and might not be able to make the 2,454 mile flight. Cockpit instruments indicated that the landing gear was stuck and couldn't be retracted. Before he could abort or continue the flight Captain Burke had to verify the information provided by the cockpit instruments. He alerted officials at Long Beach Municipal Airport (JetBlue's West Coast hub) of his situation and that he intended to fly low over the control tower to receive visual confirmation of the instrument reading. The instruments were correct. Not only was the landing gear stuck, the nose wheel had rotated ninety degrees to the left. There was no way to retract it.

Because of its long, wide runways and ample safety equipment, Captain Burke decided to try to land at Los Angeles International Airport (LAX). No landing could be considered, though, until the plane had used up most of its aviation fuel. Loaded for the cross-country flight, the A-320 can hold 46,860 pounds of fuel. That particular aircraft did not have the mechanical ability to dump fuel. The only way to get rid of it was to use it up. Less fuel reduced the risk of fire when the plane landed. It would also make the plane lighter, which would put less structural stress on the nose wheel and allow Captain Burke to come in at a slower speed.

So it was that JetBlue Flight 292 circled for hours between Bob Hope Airport and Los Angeles International Airport looping out over the Pacific Ocean while the country and even the passengers on board, thanks to the famous JetBlue Direct TV satellite service, watched the live television news coverage.

With emergency crews positioned on 11,096 foot long runway 25L, Captain Burke finally made his approach. The in flight televisions were cut off and the passengers were told to assume the heads between the knees crash positions. To keep the nose gear off the ground for as long as possible, he chose to not use reverse thrust to slow the aircraft. Because of that decision he needed almost the entire length of that very long runway. He kept the plane on its rear tires for as long as possible. When the nose gear did touch down, the resulting friction generated sparks and flames, which were quickly extinguished. Once the smoke cleared Captain Burke's spectacular landing became even more impressive. The front wheel was on the centerline of the runway.

Flight 292 ended at 6:20 that evening. Spectators gathered on buildings and stood on parked cars. Less than seven minutes later the passengers walked down the air stairs onto the tarmac with their own carry-on luggage.

The landing was smooth and there were no physical injuries. Damage to the plane was limited to tires and rims. No flights arriving at or departing from Los Angeles International Airport were delayed or cancelled. The JetBlue aircraft was repaired and returned to service still bearing the name "Canyon Blue". The flight number was changed from 292 to 358.

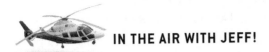

IN THE AIR WITH JEFF!

The one thing about my job that never stops amazing me is the complete unpredictability of it all. While firing the helicopter or plane up the pilot is involved with preflight details and I'm getting my 2-way radios, scanners, monitors and other equipment ready to go. It is not unusual to hear something interesting within the first few minutes.

Here's a quick aside about scanners. It took me a while to hone this skill. It's essential to know who and what to listen for—fire, police, various agencies, other news outlets and 2-way traffic all impact the area. If I just listen to a scanner that's been programmed with all the local frequencies (there are thousands in every city) I will probably miss the call "shots fired in city hall" while listening to the dog catcher in a nearby hamlet asking their dispatch if it's a white dog or a white cat. Not that dogs and cats aren't important, too, but my job is to try and keep drivers safe and unless they are in traffic I've got to keep focused on your safety.

I remember reading somewhere that it takes a minimum of 10,000 hours doing anything to be considered experienced. With 25 years on the job and still counting, I've accumulated somewhere between 50 and 60 thousand hours of flight time and airborne reporting. Even though I learn something every single day, at this point I have the experience and the confidence and know how to deal with just about any situation. I also know how to listen to a scanner.

As we were departing Van Nuys Airport to start an afternoon shift I immediately started hearing chatter on a few of my regular frequencies of something about a Jet Blue Airbus

A320 leaving nearby Bob Hope (Burbank) Airport with problems. I quickly switched around to a few others frequencies to try and confirm all this and sure enough a Jet Blue flight that departed Bob Hope was reporting that they could not retract the nose gear and were in the process of running down the procedures they have in place for such emergencies.

With that info I called the KFWB News 98 Newsroom and told them what I knew, what we were planning, and asked them to start making calls to Bob Hope, Jet Blue and any other good contacts they had. Sure enough, within minutes we were all on the same page and a drama was about to unfold over the skies of Los Angeles that would be listened to on radio, viewed on television and I think for the first time viewed by the passengers onboard Jet Blue Flight #292 via their on board Direct TV satellite televisions. They watched along with the rest of us as Los Angeles television stations started live coverage of the event.

Imagine that you're buckled into your seat just flying along and you turn on the television in the seatback in front of you to see a local television newscaster talk about a plane in trouble.

After a couple seconds you'd say, "Hey! Wait a minute. That's our plane. We're in trouble."

We started tracking the aircraft as close as possible and became the lead "Breaking News" story of the afternoon. The Jet Blue pilots were in complete control of the plane. It was not in danger while it was in the air but emergency procedures were starting to play out. The first task was to use up as much fuel as possible. This particular airliner had no fuel dump so the pilots just circled around Los Angeles, Orange County, and the Pacific Ocean just west of LAX. As we followed along, Flight 292 at one point headed for Long Beach

Airport. We thought the pilots were going to try for an emergency landing but, instead, they made a low pass over the airport so the Jet Blue engineers could get a closer look at the landing gear. They determined that right after takeoff the two wheels and tires of the nose gear had locked in a 90-degree attitude. Not only couldn't they retract into the wheel well they couldn't support any type of weight. And so the plane resumed its circling and the passengers continued watching themselves on their closed circuit seat back television screens.

We soon learned that the plane would make its emergency landing at Los Angeles International Airport's 25L runway. That's the southernmost runway at LAX and it's over two miles long. When the time for the emergency landing got close, we all got set up on the south side of LAX to wait for the aircraft.

I must say the LAX controllers were quite accommodating in letting us all work just south of one of the busiest airports in the country and with a full on emergency playing out. All the pilots of the news helicopters were following the controllers' wishes to the letter. My pilot was doing slow racetrack orbits from the ocean to the 405 freeway just south of the airport and I was narrating this whole scenario to the KFWB anchors. Our news staff was able to get officials from the FAA and Jet Blue for live interviews while this is all going on.

Finally we had the airliner in sight as it crossed the 110 freeway and approached LAX. The live running dialogue began with me from the helicopter and Tracy Savage in the studio. It was obvious to all of us that the Jet Blue pilot was going to attempt a long, slow, shallow approach. Once the main gear touched he would try to hold the nose gear off the ground as long as possible.

So here comes the jet and I'm doing this nonstop narration of what's going on as the plane gets closer and closer to the runway. These planes are big and this one's getting bigger and bigger and now I can plainly see the offending nose gear. The front wheels and tires are supposed to be straight and lined up with the runway but there're not. They are sideways. Both sides of runway 25 L are surrounded by LAX fire engines and crash crews. LA City fire is assisting. Ambulances are up and down both sides of the runway. Three helicopters from Los Angeles City circle above. County and Sheriffs' vehicles are on the ground and running. Everyone is ready for a worst-case event. The plane is over the threshold of 25L. It's getting closer to the ground and slowly, ever so slowly it seemed the main gear was on the ground. In seconds the moment we all feared would come. The nose gear would have to bear weight.

When that moment arrived the still sideways two front wheels and tires ever so gently made contact with the runway. I worried that if the front strut holding the gear snapped the plane would instantly be nose down skidding down the runway with way too many possibilities opening—way too many and none good. The nose gear held as the rubber first from one of tire and then another started to smoke. The plane, though, was still under control. It was starting to slow. The strut was still holding the nose of the aircraft up. The pilot wisely decided to not use the reverse thrusters and to just keep as much weight off the nose as possible for as long as possible.

But now the wheels themselves are dragging and sending off a brilliant shower of sparks which mixes in with the smoke from the tires. But the aircraft is still under control. Ever so slowly it rolls to a stop with no more than a thousand feet of runway left. And then the huge airplane stops.

You could almost hear the cheers from inside the plane. Now all the rescue equipment that has been racing along both sides of the runway have surrounded the plane. Water cannons and foam cannons are all deployed and ready to go. But not a single drop was needed. All 140 passengers and the 6 member crew walked or slid out of that aircraft. By the way, we later learned that the TV sets on board the plane were turned off as the landing started just to make sure all passengers would follow crew directions without the distraction of television.

Being in a situation with absolutely no input into the outcome is truly an extraordinary experience.

 ## ON THE GROUND WITH MARY!

I am a nervous flyer. To be specific, I am a nervous passenger. I don't like being buckled into a cramped seat on a commercial jet. I know thirty minutes ahead of time that we've started our descent to wherever so why did the pilot wait so long to make the announcement? My passenger nervousness isn't unusual for anyone who at one time owned and/or piloted a private airplane. When I drew up my unofficial list of things I wanted to do flying my own airplane was near the top. Decades ago I bought an old, very used Luscombe 8A and arranged to tie it down at a dirt field near my home. This little adventure might very well have been moved from the "Things-I-Want-To-Do" list to the list titled "What on earth was I thinking?". Ultimately, though, since no lives were lost

I can admit that I had a good time and learned to fly the battered Army trainer, tail dragging, squirrely plane and become a licensed pilot. I soloed, I flew cross-country, I landed before I was close enough to the ground and dropped the plane in pretty hard only to repeat the same non-landing a second time thus proving that not everyone learns as they go. The plane had no starter so I also learned to start it by spinning the propeller with all my strength. It also didn't have a gas gauge so I learned to climb on top of the cabin, open the gas cap and stick a piece of doweling down to guess how much fuel remained in the tank. It did have a compass, an artificial horizon, and an altimeter. With those instruments I could determine my direction, altitude, and whether or not I was upside down or right side up. I embraced the old saying that any landing you can walk away from is a good landing. And I also acquired the private pilot's discomfort of flying commercial. Forget that I would have absolutely no idea of how to pilot a commercial jet. Logic has no role in my discomfort.

Imagine, then, me on that Jet Blue flight circling from Bob Hope Airport out over the Pacific Ocean then back to Long Beach Airport then back to Bob Hope Airport to make the same circle over and over and over. I would have been pretty scared. I imagine that those passengers were also pretty scared.

Fear is a powerful emotion. It can inspire us to action or it can freeze us and make action impossible. Fear can create physical and emotional stress, which can lead to illness. We have unprecedented immediate access to the world around us. The news never stops. We are pummeled by world events. And it seems that the more we know the scarier life becomes. Many world events are truly scary to which our fear seems an appropriate response. However, many other events are not scary but since we are reading or hearing or viewing them through our own private lens as well as through journalistic lenses, we interpret them as scary. Our reactions to these "off the mark" interpretations are just as unhealthy as are our appropriate reactions to actual threats to our safety. Living with fear regardless of the source of the fear compromises our physical, emotional, mental and spiritual health.

Not only do we have immediate access to just about every event under the sun, we also have the ability to repeat, interpret and spread that information to everyone with whom we are connected.

Between November 2002, and July 2003, we lived in fear of SARS (Severe Acute Respiratory Syndrome). The virus started in China and spread from Hong Kong to 37 countries. It was eradicated the following year. Such potential pandemics are scary. However, in the SARS outbreak information and opinions about it spread almost faster than the virus itself.

We share and spread our fears and thus create a totally different type of pandemic. Fear is contagious. Once fear is spreading it can become, like those California wildfires, out of control. We can calm ourselves with meditation or other stress reduction techniques. We can then try, instead of spreading fear, attempting to spread calm by using the same devices with which others fuel the flames of fear. We can refuse to participate in the fear mongering.

I think I would be remiss, though, if I didn't take you a bit further into the basic cause of fear. It is a sobering discussion but I believe a necessary one.

The subject of fear boils down to this: None of us will get out of this life alive. Somewhere deep down inside we all know this fact. That may be a lot to take in but if we are to become more effective at managing our daily fears then I think we must absorb the root cause of all those other fears. Death hovers over all of us and that can feel unmanageably scary. Yet despite the fact that we live in death's shadow we must choose life every single moment of every single day if we are to truly live.

Most of the time we successfully ignore the reality of our situations. We carry on as though we are immortal. Every once in a while, though, we are reminded that life is incredibly fragile and completely unpredictable. In those moments we often embrace that which we value in life. We don't always express those values but we do on occasion acknowledge them.

In October 2002, Lt. Capt. Dimitri Kolesnikov, the commander of the Russian submarine Kursk, wrote a note to his family indicating that he and his 22 crewmates had survived the catastrophic underwater accident but acknowledged that they would die. Russian officials did not release the rest of the message because it contained a personal goodbye to the commander's family. In those moments Kolesnikov and his crew knew they would not get out of their situation alive. They got it.

On January 2, 2006, an explosion in the Sago Coal Mine trapped 13 miners for nearly two days. Only one man survived. As the men absorbed the fact that rescue was unlikely and death likely, many found scraps of paper and wrote letters to loved ones stating their love and giving assurances that death would come easily. Families reported that these letters provided comfort. In their last moments the miners understood that they would not get out of the mine alive.

Although we are not currently trapped in an unsalvageable submarine or in a collapsed tunnel of a coal mine, we are not that far removed from the sailors on the Kursk or the men trapped in the Sago Coal mine. None of us will get out of this life alive.

So where are our letters to our loved ones? Where is our appreciation of our daily miracles? Where is our gratitude? And why do we spend so much time and energy feeling afraid of something we read on social media?

Life can be scary. However, I suggest we practice threat analysis before our fight or flight survival mechanism kicks into place. Let's ask ourselves a few questions before we panic.

1. Does this information have anything to do with me?
2. Is the source of the information reliable?
3. If the information will directly impact me, what is my plan of protection?
4. Is this threat mild, serious or catastrophic?
5. Are my plans appropriate to the threat level?

Once again, let's use our heads and think things through before we panic. And let's try to not spread fear just because it's the thing to do.

President Franklin D. Roosevelt famously proclaimed that the only thing we have to fear is fear itself. Fear can rob us of the precious moments of our lives. Let's not feed it or feed on it.

Okay. That all may be easier said than done since it's coming from the person afraid of flying. Despite my fear of flying on a commercial jet, I do fly on them. Here's my secret to managing that fear and any other daily fears that come my way.

I tell myself a Japanese tale rooted in the Zen approach to life: Once upon a time a ferocious tiger chased a man. The faster the man ran the closer the tiger got to him. Finally the man ran to the edge of a cliff. He had no place to escape except over the cliff. He caught hold of a vine and swung himself over the edge and into the abyss. Dangling from the vine he looked down to the ground at least a thousand feet below him. Pacing among the boulders near the roaring waters of a river were more tigers looking up at him. The man looked back up to the cliff's edge to see if the other tiger was still there. It was staring down at him. A drop of its drool fell on his face. The man also noticed that the vine from which he hung was pulling away from the cliff's wall. He then saw a strawberry growing from the cliff next to the vine from which he hung. He knew that at any moment he would fall to his death and yet he extended one hand and picked the strawberry. As the cliff wall released the vine, the man put the strawberry into his mouth. And as he fell, the man said aloud, "What a delicious strawberry."

That is the tool with which I calm my fears. Give it a try.

THE CLOSURE OF THE 405 FREEWAY >>

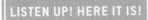

Everyone loves to hate the San Diego Freeway (The 405). Traveled by both commuters and freight haulers, the 405 is ranked as the busiest and most congested freeway in the United States. Roughly 72 miles long, Interstate 405 begins at the El Toro Y interchange with Interstate 5 in southeastern Irvine. It then runs northwest through Orange County to Long Beach in Los Angeles County. It then roughly parallels the Pacific coast for almost ten miles before crossing the Sepulveda Pass in the Santa Monica Mountains. Finally it winds through the San Fernando Valley before it ends at the 5 Freeway in Mission Hills.

The congestion problems of the 405 are legendary. During the morning and afternoon commutes the average speed on the 405 is five miles per hour. Interchanges with the Ventura Freeway (The 101) and the Santa Monica Freeway (The 10) rank among the five most congested freeway interchanges in the country. Originally designed to be a bypass route for Interstate 5, it generally takes longer to travel south or north to downtown Los Angeles using The 405 than it does taking the originally bypassed freeway, the 5.

So why do people keep using this freeway? Aside from the fact that we use it because it's there, the 405 is the only major North-South freeway between the West Los Angeles/Santa Monica areas and the areas of Downtown Los Angeles/Long Beach. It crosses the Santa Monica Mountains and connects the San Fernando Valley and the Los Angeles basin. Southern California life seems to depend on the 405 freeway.

Imagine, then, the reaction to the 2011 announcement by the California Department of Transportation (Caltrans) that for 53 hours beginning Friday night, July 15, until the following Monday morning, ten miles of the 405 between two of the nation's busiest interchanges in the Sepulveda pass would be closed. Over 250,000 vehicles pass through that pass each day. The stunned city may as well have been told that going forward there would be no air to breathe. There was no comfort as preparations began for what could only be a cataclysmic event of Biblical proportions. Without a doubt this freeway closure could only result in unprecedented traffic jams paralyzing a city and by extension the nation and doubtless by further extension the world. While local commuters might modify their schedules, tourists, with tickets purchased months before, could not. The Getty Museum would close Saturday and Sunday in the height of its season. There was no turning back, though. Preparations for the closure began.

The first order of business, therefore, was to name the closure. Lately it seems that we have to give a name to significant events. Perhaps we do this because when something has a name it seems more manageable or perhaps it hearkens back to our love of movies and all things imaginary that naming events makes them less real and therefore less frightening. For whatever reason, this freeway closure became known as "Carmageddon". Rumor has it that KNX Radio (1070 AM) created the name.

It didn't appear to matter that demolishing a bridge and rebuilding it to be more earthquake resilient was essential for safety. What mattered was that people were not going to be able to use the most hated and used freeway in the nation for one weekend.

Preparations for Carmageddon were massive. The City of Los Angeles would open its emergency operations center for that weekend. The Los Angeles Public Transit agency would provide free service on 26 bus lines and 3 of its 5 light rail lines. Caltrans asked Hollywood celebrities to warn of Carmageddon. Lady Gaga, Ashton Kutcher, Erik Estrada (possibly because people still believed he had been a member of the California Highway Patrol), warned motorists of the impending gridlock and urged them to stay off the roads the weekend of Carmageddon.

Los Angeles Mayor Antonio Villaraigosa predicted that, "It will be an absolute nightmare."

Embracing Carmageddon fever, tourist destinations from Mammoth Mountain to Las Vegas began offering special "Escape Carmageddon" discount packages. JetBlue Airways, in an "Over-the-405" promotion, offered special nonstop flights between Long Beach and Burbank for the Saturday of Carmageddon. Tickets cost $4.00 each way. Four flights would be available—two each going in either direction. When they went on sale, all 600 seats sold within three hours. Charter helicopter companies sold $150.00 air 'taxi' flights to Los Angeles International Airport from both north and south venues for travelers afraid of missing their LAX flights. Adventure Helicopter Tours offered 45-minute tours over the actual 405 closure promising a bird's eye view of not only the construction but also the traffic carnage. Champagne would be served and the tour cost $400 per person. The UCLA Medical Center obtained 600 dormitory rooms and apartments to serve as temporary quarters for hospital staff as part of an emergency plan to prevent doctors and nurses from getting stuck in traffic.

"We see this as being a disaster -- only it's a planned disaster," said Posie Carpenter, the medical center's chief administrative officer.

One month after Caltrans announced the intended closure, the dreaded weekend arrived. What had been imagined as the worst possible scenario was, in reality, nowhere near the predicted disaster. People either stayed home or took routes far away from the 405. Traffic was lighter than normal across a wide area. California Department of Transportation reported that fewer than usual vehicles were on the road. Motorists who did venture out arrived more quickly than on a normal weekend. The Metrolink commuter train system recorded its highest-ever weekend ridership since it began operating in 1991. In what became a party atmosphere in response to JetBlue's offer of special $4.00 flights between Bob Hope Airport in Burbank and Long Beach Airport, a group of cyclists challenged the jet on one of its flights. The cyclists did the same journey in one and a half hours, com-

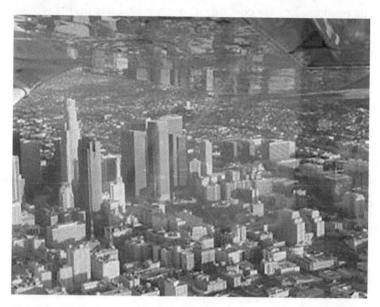

pared to two and a half hours by plane (including a drive to the airport from West Hollywood 90 minutes in advance of the flight and travel time to the end destination).

The weekend did not go by without incident, though. One man was arrested for jogging on the closed freeway. The bicyclists racing the JetBlue plane were intercepted and told to find another route. And a suspected drunk driver was arrested after going around the barricades to enter the freeway. Because people did what they were asked and the apocalyptic gridlock didn't happen there was concern that no one would pay any attention to future warnings.

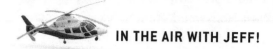

IN THE AIR WITH JEFF!

If you were told that a necessary, much used stretch of roadway in your town was going to be shut down, over a weekend . . . would you go anywhere near that area? Would you think that most of the other roads in that area might pick up the overflow? Would you make plans that perhaps for that weekend you just might stick around home? If you answered yes to all three . . . yeah, me too, along with most of the people that would drive in between the San Fernando Valley and West Los Angeles using the 405 Freeway. July 15 2011, through that weekend that's exactly what happened. The 405 freeway, the butt of many a freeway joke, comment, tale, T-shirt, license plate and other forms of endearment, the most heavily traveled and congested thoroughfare used by commuters and commerce in the country . . . would shut down to begin part of a project aimed at improving traffic flow in between West Los Angeles and the San Fernando Valley. One of many, pet peeves that I brought along from my private life in LA before becoming a traffic reporter was signage!! You're driving along, probably a tad late, and you're approaching the exit you need to continue your commute, only to find as you get close, a sign that proclaims. . . ."NEXT EXIT CLOSED," meaning of course THIS EXIT!! Didn't that just light you up!!! Does for me!! So, the next step in this adventure that you never wanted, is to follow the rest of the cattle to the next exit, probably way off your intended path and sit in the back up with everyone else waiting to get off at some mysterious exit that you never use. Wow! Thankfully this practice is starting to change but more on that later. The thought should be, start placing the little portable sign that says . . . "whatever is closed" 2 or 3 exits BEFORE the actual closure thereby giving you an option or two!! I'm no highway engineer but I think that might help you a bit. So, back to "Carmageddon!!" What made the difference with this adventure was the press releases from Caltrans and Metro warning of this closures months in advance.

This time, they put the sign way in advance of the closure.

Los Angles radio, television, print, social media, Twitters and Bloggers all jumped on the pending disaster and forecast of peril, chaos and doom. First responders set up contingency plans for getting to areas within the closure. County Supervisors and other city and state officials made comments through media outlets urging residents to stay home that weekend. Plans for getting staff in and out of crucial places like hospitals, government offices, University of California at Los Angeles (UCLA) and others on the West Side were drawn up. Some police jurisdictions that had personnel that normally would commute through that area made plans to stay at their postings all weekend. Residents of Malibu braced for what seemed like a pending onslaught of traffic driving between Ventura and Santa Monica using little 2 lane Pacific Coast Highway.

This time they really put the signs up way in advance of the closure and it worked! The Friday evening of the beginning of the closure is at hand. We are flying back and forth in between LAX (Los Angeles International Airport) and the San Fernando Valley over the 405 and all the surface streets of West Los Angeles (which, by the way are jammed every day of the week, without "Carmageddon.") Around 3:00 pm things look quite normal-busy to me. The studio keeps asking "Are things getting crazy out there yet?" "Nope, still looks ok to me." Before I go further I should explain to you if you don't live in or have never visited Los Angeles, the terms *okay, normal, predictable,* or *civilized* when describing traffic have different meanings from their meanings in most other cities. Take the term *"Civilized"*. It's a favorite of mine. Drivers who have been listening to me for years know and trust the description to mean, perhaps a ten mile stretch of freeway during the 5:00 PM hour, from this interchange to that interchange is slow but moving for the most part, maybe a touch of stop and go but there are no lanes blocked for whatever reason and "You should be okay!" So, that's how West Los Angeles traffic is looking this particular afternoon going into the now infamous "Carmageddon" weekend in Los Angeles. The about to shut down 405 is okay. The West Los Angeles surface streets are normal, quite busy and I've had no Godzilla or RoDan sightings!

The 405 shuts down later that evening. Other freeways do not become parking lots, surface streets do not gridlock, everything looks okay. The reason for this closure was the dismantling of the Mulholland Bridge that spans the 405 at the top of what's called the Sepulveda Pass. It's a huge undertaking by the construction crews that have promised to complete the job in time to reopen the 405 for the Monday morning commute. For the rest of that weekend radio, television and social media would document every jackhammer, pick, ripped rebar, concrete chunks of what was once a bridge falling to the ground and into waiting trucks to be carried away. Between construction noise, helicopters and other aircraft and news crews on scene, the residents of the nearby neighborhoods had a rather tiring weekend. Traffic, oh that was fine. Remember, they got that "Signage thing" right this time!

We flew all weekend through the daylight hours. Earlier I said traffic was fine through these events but that's not quite accurate. During "Carmageddon II" there was a planned but seemingly forgotten (in the shadow of Carmageddon) event that really put the squeeze on surface streets in-between Venice and downtown Los Angeles. The 2012 Los Angles triathlon made it quite difficult to cross east/west surface streets to allow the bicyclists section of the triathlon to bike from Venice towards Staples center. Plus, wait: There is more to these memorable weekends in Los Angeles. The 2012 Cirque du Soleil show "Iris," secured a permit to close the intersection of Hollywood Blvd. and Highland Avenue Saturday morning through Monday night!

Okay, pull out the Thomas Guide for Los Angeles, turn to pages 632 and 633, which shows you most of Los Angeles, west of down town and finally pull out as many different colored magic markers you own. Ready? First draw a red line over the 405 from the 1-10 Santa Monica Freeway to the I-10/405 interchange in Encino-Sherman Oaks. Next draw a red line over Venice Blvd. near the beach all the way into downtown Los Angeles. Almost done. Now yellow lines over Olympic, Fairfax and Hope. One could not drive the red lines, or in the case of Venice and Olympic cross the red line! These closures and rolling closures were to be in place from around 7:00 AM through noon Saturday. It was an adventure to get from let's say UCLA to LAX for a good part of Saturday. Okay, maybe I did glimpse Rodan coming in over the Pacific once or twice but he never made it and we all survived. I was interviewed by stations as far away as Arizona trying to have fun with the Los Angeles traffic phenomena of "Carmageddon." We did somewhat but the bottom line was that most people made plans to not drive around the impacted areas for the weekend and the "Signage" was put out way in advance, way before the closure. You knew BEFORE leaving home that weekend where not to drive. Well done!

ON THE GROUND WITH MARY!

The weekend closure of a section of the 405 Freeway did not stop a city. We were warned and for the most part we paid attention to the warnings. Life changed somewhat for 72 hours or so and then life routinely resumed. Did we get all worked up and excited? Of course. That's what we humans tend to do. We doubtless felt anxious and we worried and perhaps we even stockpiled paper towels and toothpaste just in case. We did, however, survive. The adrenaline rush slowed and our blood pressure returned to its dangerously high normal level. We didn't know what life would be like with the closure of part of the 405 so even if we don't ordinarily use that freeway we experienced anxiety.

One day I was stuck in traffic on the 405 but, then, what else is new? We've all been stuck there at one time or another either actually or metaphorically. On this particular day, though, I was stuck behind a bus. There was no way around the bus. Vehicles on both sides of me were also stuck. I don't know why we are all sitting there going nowhere. Sometimes that's just how it is. Anyway, I was sitting there in my car breathing bus exhaust fumes and staring at a sign on the back of the bus.

"Happiness Is An Inside Job."

That's what the sign said and as I drummed my fingers on the steering wheel it occurred to me that all of our thoughts and emotions are inside jobs. So there it is. Just like happiness, anxiety is an inside job. We don't have to feel it. The choice is ours.

However, before we can manage our anxiety we should probably first find out its address. Most of us have some sort of address that we call home. It might not be the address of our dreams but we do have some place to go at the end of the day. For many of us that home address is different from the home address of our childhoods. And for those of us hoping to make a move, our current home address isn't the address for which we hope. Most of us, though, do have a current address. For those among us who have multiple homes, that's okay. You can still play along because I'm thinking that regardless of how many homes you have you can only be in one at a time.

For example –

1. Where did you live when you were a child?

....

2. Where would you like to live in three years?

....

3. Where are you right now (which home are you in)?

....

By the way, if all of the addresses are the same you might actually be a truly contented person. But supposing they aren't, what would happen if you went back to the address of your childhood, knocked on the door, and announced that you were home for dinner? If your family still lives there, this probably won't be a shock to anyone but if strangers are currently living there, you might have some explaining to do because their home is no longer your home. And imagine that you arrive at the home in which you hope to live in three years. You knock on the door and announce that you're home for dinner and the people have never seen you before. Again, you'll have some explaining to do. We understand, then, that we can't actually be in three places at the same time nor can we live in the home of our past nor in the home of our future. We're stuck right here in the present.

Just as our physical selves have locations, so do our emotions and they are the same locations: The Past. The Future. The Present.

List a couple of things about which you currently worry or feel anxious:

1. I worry about ....

2. I worry about ....

3. I worry about ....

Now, where do all those worries live? In the past, the present or the future? Worry and anxiety live in the future. When we worry about the 405 being closed or feel anxious about whether or not we should stockpile paper towels and toothpaste we are trying to outsmart or control the future. It's really hard to just sit with uncertainty. We want to do something about it so we try to control it even though we know that is impossible. Even with the best precautions, the future cannot be known. In our attempts to control we feel nervous or anxious. We worry.

We may think we also feel anxious or worry about the past but that's not really possible. The past is over. There's no going back. That's doesn't keep us from trying, though. Guilt or regret or shame keep guiding us back not to control the past but to change it. That, also, is a pointless endeavor. So what have we left to us? The only thing we ever had was the present.

Unfortunately our anxiety and our regret create quite a bit of stress and that stress makes it much more difficult for us to enjoy the only thing we ever had to begin with. Stress can rob us of the present. Stress also takes a toll on us emotionally, behaviorally, and physically.

Let's take a minute to examine the source of our stress. Check off any that apply to you.

- I worry about the economy and/or my own finances.
- I worry about my job performance.
- I worry about how long my car will hold up.
- I worry about traffic and my commute.
- I worry about the ache in my shoulder.
- I worry about my weight.
- I worry about at least one member of my family.
- I worry about growing old.
- I worry about my health.

Now listen up. If you checked one item or more, you must be human. We all worry and we all feel anxious. We read about the harmful impact of prolonged stress and yet we continue to feed it. Where does stress live? It lives in the future because with our worry and anxiety we are trying to control the future.

Right about now I suggest you consider whether your primary emotional address is in the past or the future or the present. Where do your feelings spend most of their time? I'm thinking that, like all of us, you spend way too much time trying to change the past or manage the future. With practice you can change your primary emotional residence to the present. We'll talk more about ways of spending more emotional time in the present but for now please just consider submitting a change of address form to yourself and make your home base the present—the here and now.

THE GLENDALE METROLINK TRAIN CRASH

LISTEN UP! HERE IT IS!

Early on the morning of January 26, 2005, Juan Manuel Alvarez left his Jeep Cherokee on the railroad tracks near a crossing just south of Chevy Chase Drive in Glendale, California. At 6:03 that same morning the southbound Metrolink commuter train #100 struck the Jeep causing it to derail and veer right onto a siding where a Union Pacific locomotive was parked. Metrolink #100 hit the locomotive, which caused its first two cars to jackknife just as the northbound Metrolink #901 was passing. The cars from the #100 jackknifed into the #901 between its second and third car, causing the third car to fall onto its side.

The impacts sent passengers flying through the train cars. Several cars caught fire. Eleven people died and more than 200 were injured. For the next three years this would be the deadliest incident in Metrolink history. At the time it was also the deadliest train wreck in United States history.

Alvarez was arrested in a nearby hospital while being treated for self-inflicted cuts to his chest and arm. He had apparently cut himself after the crash.

He told hospital staff, "It's my fault."

Identified by witnesses who saw him running away from his Jeep, Mr. Alvarez was arrested and charged with 11 counts of first-degree murder with the special circumstances of multiple murder.

As he was arrested he was heard muttering, "I'm sorry. I'm sorry."

Authorities and the legal defense team for Mr. Alvarez claimed that he had been planning on committing suicide by blocking the tracks so the train could hit him while he sat in his Jeep. At the last minute he changed his mind and abandoned the vehicle. In 2008 he was convicted to 11 consecutive life sentences with no possibility of parole.

Thirty-five ambulances responded along with nearly 300 firefighters from Glendale, Los Angeles, Pasadena and Ventura. They were joined by a Hazmat team. Uninjured passengers also became first responders as they assisted each other from the wreckage. First responders also included employees of a nearby Costco who climbed fences to offer blankets and bottled water.

 IN THE AIR WITH JEFF!

Our shift started out like most winter mornings in LA, dark, damp and a lot of clouds that created low ceilings here and there. We have just flown out of the San Fernando Valley by transitioning east along the 101/134 freeways out of Van Nuys airspace and through Burbank's airspace that has just cleared us to the south via the I-5 or Golden State Freeway. My pilot is Adam Bennett, an experienced and seasoned media pilot. Adams is fun to be with and we are joking about what the hell we're doing flying around Los Angeles at this hour in this weather! The scanner has been blurting out a fair amount of stuff in the short time we've been flying until one of those dispatches hits.

I hear a call from the LAPD Hot Shot channel for a call on, "Car on tracks and on fire."

It went on a bit, but this is one of those dispatches that you chase down fast. It mentioned a Metrolink/Union Pacific track and a Glendale street. That's Glendale Police Department territory so it all added to the bit of urgency to my ears. About a minute after I hear this, I tell Adam and ask him to do a 180-degree fast and get up to the location. We were over the 110/I-5 interchange near Dodger Stadium at the moment and the call was just a mile or two north of us near Chevy Chase Drive. Remember that my main responsibility is traffic reporting and in about thirty seconds I hear the station's intro hit for traffic. Jack Popejoy and Judy Ford were the KFWB anchors at the time.

All of a sudden I hear Jack say with the traffic jingle, "Six eleven. It's time for traffic on the ones. Here's Rhonda Kramer."

Rhonda was our morning traffic anchor. Rhonda does a few incidents and then throws to me. I do something on a minor incident on the Golden State Freeway and then mention that I'm hearing about a possible car fire near the Metrolink tracks in Glendale. I add that we're just a minute away.

I sign off with "Stick with us. More to follow."

Adam has now gotten us almost over the incident in Glendale. We're flying low under this low cloud ceiling over the tracks that run north-south through Glendale and in between Chevy Chase Drive and Los Feliz Boulevard. Now I have switched my 2 way over to the KFWB news frequency and off air tell the editor that I'm here and it's real bad. Then still off the air I tell him, "Come to me. I'm ready."

Within a heartbeat I hear Jack Popejoy on the air introducing me. "If you listened to our last traffic report you heard Jeff mention something about a possible car fire on railroad tracks. Jeff what do you see?"

That line would set off about six hours of the most intense airborne reporting I think I have ever done or ever will do. All of the critical factors for us were bad. Adam has skillfully flown us right where we need to be so I can see the event. It's dark. There's a low ceiling. Power lines are all over the place. Now a TV ship has heard the same thing I did and they are inbound. It hasn't even started yet and the tension gauge is pinned in the red!

As I look out my left side window, through the clouds, straining my eyeballs to the max I reply to Jack and our listeners, "Something really bad has happened here. We're circling over the Metro tracks that run through Glendale just south of Chevy Chase Drive. Something happened to cause a train to --oh dear -- now I can see a car or two that have jackknifed and possibly hit a train going the other direction. Flames are visible to me now. It's just next to the Costco in Glendale. There are lots of flashlights visible. People coming out of the warehouse. (We are doing sort of an oblong race-track shaped orbit over this scene so every new angle presents something new to me.) Be careful I see Glendale Fire pulling into the parking lot and I've heard Los Angeles City Fire responding too. Oh here they come now. Be careful if you're driving on Los Feliz Boulevard. A lot of fire equipment is responding to the scene here. There's more police arriving. I think Glendale PD is racing down Central. If you're just joining us be so very careful driving in Glendale. There are fire and police from Glendale and Los Angeles arriving from all directions to San Fernando Road just south of Chevy Chase Drive. Wherever I look I can see flashing red lights coming this way. Please be careful driving. Jack, I think I can see one car of this Metrolink is on its side and I think something else has happened just north of here on the tracks.

There are about three engine companies working a few hundred yards to the north."

Wherever I looked it was madness, more TV ships arrived, the airspace was jammed as well but the level of cooperation was extraordinary. I thought Adams head was going to spin off his neck as he avoided possible mid-air collisions. It was a target rich environment to say the least! The commentary between Jack, Judy and me was almost nonstop. We were into this and completely out of the news clock or format going through twenty minutes now. At one point my 2 way just overheated and quit but thankfully recovered. Jack Popejoy and Judy Ford could now see some of the TV footage and were asking me really intelligent questions.

As we are doing this I have the scanner still running at a low level in my left ear and all I can hear is, "This company. That company. Car this. Car that. Rescue ambulance so and so. Glendale Fire and LA City Fire respond to . . . "

The separate incident just north of the train is now getting a lot of attention from Fire and Police. Ever so slowly, it seemed to take forever but daylight would reveal the magnitude of the tragedy.

Finally, as daylight came and the low clouds cleared a bit it wasn't too hard to tell what had happened. It looked like the southbound Metrolink train hit an SUV that was parked on the tracks a little south of Chevy Chase Drive. The train continued south but then the lead car of 4 (It was in the pusher mode with the engine in the back.) derailed and in a worst-case scenario where there was a stretch of three parallel sets of tracks to accommodate other trains, crashed into a side-lined freight car and a passing northbound Metrolink train on the other track! It just couldn't have happened in a tighter spot.

Our day continued till about 1:00 pm when the station finally released us. The story and tragedy continued for days, weeks and months after that. Eventually we would all learn that the vehicle I had noticed and mentioned in all the chaos of that dark, misty, overcast, tragic morning just north of where the train came to rest was the cause of the incident. A man had tried to commit suicide but had a change of heart as the train approached and jumped out of the SUV but left it on or near the tracks. Eleven people died. Almost 200 were injured. It involved the resources of the Glendale/Pasadena Fire departments, the Los Angeles City and County Fire Departments, the Los Angeles Police Department, the Glendale Police Department and countless other first responders and some unsung heroes. Some of the early employee arrivals at Costco were actually the first on scene, running out of their store and climbing over a chain link fence to help. The person who left the car on the tracks was tried for 11 counts of murder, found guilty and is now serving 11 consecutive life sentences with no possibility of parole.

 ON THE GROUND WITH MARY!

This Glendale train wreck was truly traumatic. There is no denying that. A traumatic event in many ways resembles the pebble tossed into the pond. To one degree or another that pebble hitting the water impacts and changes everything. The greatest impact is on the pebble and the immediate water into which it was tossed. Then the ripple effect starts with diminishing intensity relative to the distance from the point of impact.

Those most significantly impacted by this event were, of course, those people on the train, the first responders including the Costco employees, and those who directly witnessed the tragedy. Impacted by the ripples were all of us who heard about it on the radio or read about it in the newspapers or saw the images aired relentlessly on television. Those who reported the event, including our own Jeff Baugh, were also touched by the trauma ripples. And, of course, those whose loved ones (family and friends) were injured or killed were so close to the event that they, too, experienced significant effects of trauma.

I define trauma as any event that throws our universe into chaos. That's a pretty broad definition but I like it because we all react differently to different events. In our lives we can reasonably expect to experience at least one potential traumatic event. Some of us experience far more potentially traumatic events. I say potential because the same event is not necessarily traumatic for everyone impacted. We are all different in our resilience, in our coping mechanisms, and in our worldviews. How we react to the events of our lives is as different as are we different from all of the people in our lives.

The modern study of how trauma impacts human functioning began after the Vietnam War and for the first time we heard the term "Post Traumatic Stress Disorder" to describe cognitive, emotional and behavioral changes related to a specific psychiatric diagnosis. Such a diagnosis refers to maladaptive thoughts, feelings, and actions and generally requires professional interventions. However, even without a diagnosis, we all respond to trauma uniquely and individually.

Because of our unprecedented access to information we are bombarded with actual and vicarious potential trauma reactions on an almost constant basis. Even if the ripples don't touch us we know the event happened and that knowledge impacts our view of the world. We begin to feel less safe in our home environments even if the event took place thousands of miles away.

There's an obvious and fairly simple solution to some of our vicarious experiences of traumatic events. We can at least stop reading the social media postings, which all too often graphically and inaccurately portray these events. We can choose reliable news sources to read, listen to or view and avoid those that sensationalize the news.

While we can control to a certain extent our vicarious trauma exposure, so much of what happens in our lives is beyond our control. We will experience trauma and our universe will feel chaotic and out of control. To regain stability and equilibrium we must discover and employ methods of normalizing the traumatic event. How is it possible, you doubtless ask, to normalize a shooting or a train wreck or an act of terrorism or even the loss of a loved one?

I absolutely do not mean that we should decide that these aren't extraordinary, horrible tragedies but are normal life events. There is nothing normal or every day about a train wreck and we don't ever want such an event to become part of our daily experience. By normalizing I mean that one way to help us with our response to trauma is to incorporate the event into our life narrative. By doing so our universe can begin to regain order. Our planets can resume their orbits. Their orbits may be slightly changed but the sense of chaos will diminish.

Without some sort of reclamation of order in our lives we may begin to exhibit symptoms of distress either physically or psychologically or behaviorally. Such symptoms might include disturbing dreams about the event, avoiding people or places or activities that remind us of the event. We might not be able to recall details of the event or even the actual event itself. We might blame ourselves for it. We might persistently feel fear or anger or guilt or shame. We might display irritation or anger. We might start behaving recklessly or engage in self-destructive behavior. We might have difficulty concentrating or be always on the alert to the point that we are easily startled. We might experience disturbances of sleep or appetite. Experiencing or exhibiting a few of those symptoms is normal and expectable. Get ready for them. However, if what you are thinking or feeling or doing is making it more difficult for you to function—to get through the day— then you might consider getting some professional guidance.

Research indicates that there are things you can do to help speed along your trauma recovery, minimize your discomfort, and help you restore order to your chaotic universe. A presentation at a British Psychology Society conference proposed that engaging in the seemingly trivial task of playing the video game Tetris diminished symptoms associated with a traumatic event. Further research supports that proposal. Focusing on an engaging visual-spatial task may significantly reduce our trauma symptoms. It seems that the less time between the event and Tetris the more effectively we respond to the benefits of the game. I have observed first responders take a break and start playing Tetris on their phones. Tetris is no cure all nor is it an instant fix if we are already experiencing stress related symptoms. And it may not be the only such activity available. It does, however, indicate that we can utilize the neuroplasticity of our brains to avoid the deep ruts of the traumatic event.

Video games aren't the only way to minimize the effects of

exposure to trauma. Talking about our experiences or writing about them may also hold powerful healings. Unfortunately, we all too often keep silent. We are possibly afraid or ashamed to share our experiences or to even put them in writings read only by ourselves. Sometimes the sharing of our trauma stories is even considered taboo. This appears to be an especially accurate observation in the military or sports cultures in which at least appearing to be mentally tough, competitive, and physically impenetrable seems essential. The vocabulary of war—whether military or sports—has no words for expressions of vulnerability. And so our warriors and our sports heroes, too, often have no words for their trauma. Since we are lovers of military and athletic combat we tend to model our behaviors upon that of our heroes and are thus also rendered silent in the face of trauma. Eventually the impact of trauma takes its toll. It's far healthier to break the taboo of silence than to suffer in silence. Perhaps we all would benefit from remedial courses focused on the language of pain. With words we create and with words we heal.

A woman whose husband was killed in the mass shootings at the Virginia Polytechnic Institute and State University (Virginia Tech) shared that she felt silenced by the emotional imprint of her trauma. Through writing she regained emotional control and was eventually able to reclaim her very changed life.

Whether what we write about our trauma experience is read by anyone else doesn't much matter. It's the writing that helps us heal. Talking about our experiences, however, requires a listener. Research in organizational psychology indicates that social support reduces the impact of trauma. We get it that social support is important in any situation. Unfortunately, a traumatic event can scatter or render inaccessible our social support system. Throughout this book we've encouraged you to list people you can turn to, activities that sustain you, and things for which you are grateful. Trauma makes it all the more important to keep those lists you made throughout this book accessible always but especially in cases of emergency.

Traumatic events happen either to us or around us. With time, attention, and support we can reduce the chaos and reclaim a new life coherency. Please don't be afraid or ashamed to reach out for help and support. We are all in this together. The very least we can do is assist each other.

THE CHATSWORTH TRAIN WRECK

Trains are enormous. A crashing train releases devastating force. It becomes unmanageable and unstoppable. Passengers can do nothing to prevent carnage from happening. They are often tossed around inside the cars. Broken limbs, internal injuries, and death are expected consequences of train collisions or derailments.

On September 13, 2008, at 4:30 PM PST in the Chatsworth area of the San Fernando Valley north of Los Angeles a freight train collided with a rush-hour commuter train. The force of the collision was so intense that an engine from the freight train lodged into a Metrolink passenger car. The locomotive of the Metrolink commuter train 111 weighed 250,000 pounds. It pulled three Bombardier Bi-level Coaches and 222 people were aboard when it collided head-on with an eastbound Union Pacific local freight train. Two SD0ACe locomotives weighing 408,000 pounds each pulled the 17 freight cars. The Metrolink locomotive telescoped backward into the passenger compartment of the first passenger car and caught fire. All three locomotives, the leading Metrolink passenger car and ten freight cars, were derailed and both lead locomotives and the passenger car toppled over.

Both trains were on the same section of single track that runs between the Chatsworth Station (which is double tracked) through the Santa Susana Pass. The line returns to double track again as it enters the Simi Valley. This single-track section carries 24 passenger trains and 12 freight trains each day. The line's signaling system is designed to ensure that trains wait on the double track section while a train is proceeding in the other direction on the single track. The Metrolink train would normally wait in the Chatsworth station for the daily Union Pacific freight train to pass before proceeding. Both trains were moving toward each other at the time of the collision. At least one passenger on the Metrolink train saw the freight train moments before impact, coming around the curve. The freight train's engineer triggered the emergency air brake only two seconds before impact, while the Metrolink engineer never applied the brakes on his train.

Originally the Los Angeles Fire Department dispatched a single engine company with a four-person crew for a "possible physical rescue" at a residential address near the scene in response to an emergency call from the home. The crew arrived at the address four minutes later and cut through the backyard fence to evaluate the situation. The captain on the scene immediately called for an additional five ambulances, then 30 fire engines, and after reaching the wreck he called for every heavy search and rescue unit in the city. Hundreds of emergency workers were eventually involved in the rescue and recovery efforts, including 250 firefighters. Two Los Angeles city firefighters received medals for risking their lives to enter a confined space without their air bottles to rescue one of the freight train engineers.

The National Transportation Safety Board (NTSB) investigated the cause of the collision, and concluded that the Metrolink train ran through a red signal before entering a section of single track where the opposing freight train had been given the right of way. The NTSB faulted the Metrolink train's engineer for the collision, concluding that he was distracted by text messages he was sending to teenage train enthusiasts while on duty. Robert M. Sanchez, who died in the crash seconds after sending his last text message, apparently failed to obey a red stop signal that indicated it was not safe to proceed into the single track section of the route.

A total of 25 people died in the collision including engineer Sanchez and two victims who died at hospitals in the days following the crash. This event became the deadliest railway accident in Metrolink's history, and one of the deadliest in the United States.

A total of 135 others were reported injured, 46 of them critically, with 85 of the injured transported to 13 hospitals and two transported themselves. Los Angeles Fire Department Captain Steve Ruda reported that the high number of critically injured passengers taxed the area's emergency response capabilities, and patients were distributed to all 12 trauma centers in Los Angeles County.

The four other crewmembers of the two trains survived. The conductor and engineer of the freight train were trapped inside the lead locomotive while it was engulfed in flames; the firefighters who rescued the pair found them banging on the thick glass windshield, unable to escape. One of the passengers who died in this crash was a survivor of the 2005 Glendale train crash.

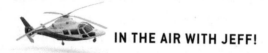 **IN THE AIR WITH JEFF!**

I'm sure by now you've got it that listening to a scanner can give a first alert of something going on, that might be of interest to an airborne reporter. You get used to hearing a Fire Department or Police dispatch, and in my world, the California Highway Patrol (CHP), Caltrans, and the like. They are all straight forward and usually will sound somewhat predictable. For instance, a fire dispatch will instruct the engine companies to respond to a report of fire at so and so location and give a brief description of the reported fire. From that point the requested engines will go to that location and report what they see—a fire, maybe just a bit of smoke, nothing, or they will investigate and advise. Police dispatches are similar except the call goes out for the report of a crime or help requested and any unit close will pick up the call and respond. Police departments are out cruising. Fire departments are based at stations and respond to calls. You have to be heads up and use experience to decide which ones to check out in the "dispatch" phase. If you know what you're doing, a helicopter with a savvy pilot and crew can sometimes get on scene before or just as first responders arrive. On the way you give your newsroom a heads up that you're going to check something out and either it's a story or it's not. So, it's always the unusual call that should get your undivided attention.

On a September afternoon while flying over Los Angeles City Hall chasing down a traffic incident, I heard one of those calls. It was a LAPD Hot Shot call for a dispatch to an address in Chatsworth.

Someone was reporting that there was "a train on their front lawn!" You can bet the farm that got my attention! Didn't matter to me if it wound up being bogus or not. We were going to check this one out. This particular day was the first shift I was flying with a pilot named Dan Rudert. Dan and fellow pilot Cliff Fleming had recently made national news as the pilots of the Helicopter Retrieval Operation of the Genesis Space Probe for NASA. The bottom line for me was that I was in good hands. I asked Dan to get us in the general direction of Topanga Canyon and the 118 freeway FAST and I'd guide us in from there. When the "in the traffic" report came up I mentioned that I was heading into the San Fernando Valley to check out a report of a possible train incident with more to follow.

By now we are over Paramount Studios and Dan is peeling the paint off of Jet Copter 98 heading towards Chatsworth. The situation was ramping up very quickly! I'm now talking to the news desk at KFWB. They are telling me that indeed they are getting calls to the newsroom from listeners reporting something happening on the Metro tracks in Chatsworth. We are now at warp speed coming over the Encino reservoir heading to the Metro tracks just east of Topanga Canyon. The pilot has us cleared through Van Nuys airport airspace and now I can hear on the helicopter comms that TV ships based at Van Nuys Airport are heading to the same event.

It was at that instant I heard the defining call on the scanner from the LA City Fire Engine Company that had the original dispatch saying to "Send everything we have!"

It was the voice of an almost breathless fire fighter on scene! The next 15 or so minutes were a blur. We are now in an orbit over Chatsworth, south of the 118 freeway, east of Stony Point (a popular climbing area) and looking at a jumbled mess of train cars just out of one of tunnel where the tracks turn south towards the Chatsworth station. I'm describing what I see, the trains—the small fire which is already going out, railroad cars on their sides, fire personnel now putting ladders up against the car on its side trying to evacuate riders from the windows that are pointing skyward, fire personnel and police responding from all directions to a difficult-to-get-to-spot. The media pilots are doing an extraordinary job of talking to each other and keeping us all separated.

Below us more and more first responders arrive. It looks like Los Angeles County Fire has been asked to assist and the scanner traffic is getting more and more solemn. There is the chatter of possible fatalities inside the trains. It goes on for about 10 or 15 minutes of nonstop talk between me and the KFWB anchors—them asking questions and me doing my best to answer them. I still have the scanner up in one of my ears when I just halted for a few seconds. It took those few seconds to process what I was seeing. Finally I was able to get it out of my brain and into my voice.

"It looks like there's been a head-on crash just outside of the tunnel with the engine of one train actually penetrating the passenger car of the other!"

Sadly this was not the last of trains versus other trains, cars, trucks or people. I found it odd on my arrival in Los Angeles at the lack of widespread public transportation available in the late 1970's. Growing up in a large east coast city, it was a normal way of life taking above ground light rail (AKA the trolley), subways and buses to school or anywhere one needed to go. I'm told that turn-of-the-century Los Angeles did have lots of light rail but falling in love with freeways, cars, cheap gasoline, suburban housing and the freedom of instant gratification when it came to travel put public transportation on the back burner for a long time.

Covering as many of these train vs. train vs. whatever incidents through the years has led me to believe that Los Angeles drivers and even pedestrians never really learned how to co-exist with trains. You can't beat the train to the crossing. You can't walk along busy railroad tracks. You can stop a car or truck much faster than an engineer can stop a train. If the other side of the train crossing is backed up, don't try to get to the tracks. You get the idea I'm sure. But it seems that these terrible things happen every day in and around Los Angeles. We must learn how to better live with trains. With the new light rail service that is now expanding in Los Angeles and connecting so many neighborhoods, it's never been more important.

I just want to add one postscript to the day I flew over the Chatsworth train tragedy. Later that year I was awarded a Golden Mike by the Radio and Television News Association for my coverage of that disaster. I had a duplicate trophy made for Dan Rudert with a special plaque installed on the base thanking him for his brilliant work that day. He was thrilled. So was I.

 ## ON THE GROUND WITH MARY!

Investigation revealed that the engineer was texting while in charge of his train. Regardless of how convinced we are that we can do two things at once, we can't. Multi-tasking is a myth. Chances are this engineer didn't mean to cause one of the worst accidents in railroad history nor did he mean for people and himself to die. Nevertheless the accident happened and people died because Robert Sanchez wasn't paying attention to his one and only responsibility.

We live distracted lives. Phones ring. Text messages arrive. Email messages demand response. Our televisions provide thousands of viewing choices for simultaneous viewing. Social media invites us to watch videos of kittens riding robotic vacuum cleaners or beagles used for cosmetic testing first stepping onto real grass. And still meals must be selected or prepared. Clothes must be washed and bills must be paid which reminds us that somewhere we do something to earn our livings. We live very complicated lives.

As the poet Emily Dickenson observed, "To live is so startling, it leaves but little room for other occupations . . .".

Her observation implies that our most important occupation is to live. We would propose that we not strive to live lives of misery but lives of meaning embracing optimism and tranquility. Such a life demands attention.

Paying attention to just one thing at a time can seem impossible. Maintaining focus is just something the adventure action hero does in the film's most exciting moments. If we are to survive the day and enjoy some level of inner contentment, we must learn to focus and pay attention to just one thing at a time. We must learn to become mindful of the moment.

We are not in the habit of giving our attention to the mundane activities of our lives. We go about our days almost in a mindless state. We drive as though we are in a trance paying little attention to the road or the other vehicles. We trip and we spill because of inattention. A friend says something to us and we forget what was said almost as soon as the words are out of his or her mouth. We eat unaware that we are doing so. We don't notice the signals we receive from our bodies that we are tired or in discomfort. We worry about the past or the future.

Becoming mindful does not require that we abandon life to go live on a mountain and spend our days meditating in quiet and solitude. With mindful living we still pay the bills and go to work and wash the clothes and clean the house. Becoming mindful only requires that we learn to pay attention with focus and without judgment. Whatever we do we give our full attention. The laundry receives our full attention. Because our focus is on the present task we are not able to worry about the past, the future, or even other tasks in the present because our complete attention is on the task at hand.

The only moment we have is this very moment. The past is gone. The future is not guaranteed. Our precious moments quickly pass by us. Practicing mindfulness can help us slow those moments down and calm our hectic lives, minds, and spirits.

It's simple to search mindfulness exercises. I'm going to give you a few suggestions but you can identify or create many more that will be equally helpful.

My first suggestion is that you simply sit down and focus on your breathing. Don't try to control it. Don't try to change it. Just pay attention to it. If your thoughts drift from your breathing to your list of daily tasks without condemnation bring them back to your breathing. Spend a moment or two in this state of awareness.

You might also give this a try. Sit in a kitchen or dining room chair. Put both feet on the floor. Try to relax your entire body. If you are comfortable doing so, close your eyes. Just sit and pay attention first to what you feel physically. Do you feel the back of the chair against your own back? Do you feel the edge of the chair on your legs? Do you feel the collar of your shirt against the back of your neck? What about your hair? Can you feel it touching your face at all? Take stock of these sensations for a while. When you've accounted for just about all that you are feeling physically, switch your attention to what you are hearing or smelling. Did a truck just drive by? Did you hear it? What about footsteps outside your apartment? Is your neighbor next door or down the hall baking bread again? Isn't that the most amazing thing to smell? Give your attention to these auditory and olfactory sensations until you've had enough.

How was that for you? Take a moment and just jot down your reflections on those experiences.

....

....

....

....

The value of this exercise is that giving our physical and our sensory experiences our full attention leaves little if any room for thought.

Since we tend to eat on the run and often with little awareness of what or how much we are eating, you might also give a try to some mindful eating. It doesn't really matter what you eat when you try this. You could mindfully eat your peanut butter and jelly sandwich or your afternoon apple or your morning pancakes. Just for the sake of discussion, let's have you eat your afternoon apple. Hold it in your hand. Take a careful look at it. What color is it? Is it a solid color or does the skin have variations in color? Is the stem still attached? Hold it up into the light and see what else you can observe. Before taking your first bite, decide where, exactly, you are going to bite into the apple. Wow! That might be a tough one. Once you made that decision, go ahead and take a first, small bite. Don't try to eat the whole apple in one bite. There's no need for that. Now you've got a piece of apple in your mouth. Take time to experience the taste of it and the feel of it before you start chewing. And when you do start chewing, chew slowly.

If you've actually put down this book and eaten an apple, reflect here on the experience.

. . . .

. . . .

. . . .

. . . .

. . . .

When a friend or family member talks to you, really listen. All too often we are planning our response instead of hearing the words spoken by the other person. Try to not respond until you are certain the other person has finished speaking.

Try listing the things in life for which you are grateful. The list can include people, body parts, hobbies, automobiles, health, and good books—anything for which you feel a sense of appreciation or gratitude. Give that a try right now. List 3 things for which you are grateful.

1. . . . .

2. . . . .

3. . . . .

Another list you might find useful is a list of activities, people, or things that leave you feeling happy. These list making activities help us focus on and give our attention to activities that require thought and crowd out worries and anxieties.

You have just taken some beginning steps toward mindfulness. With mindfulness we can reclaim calm and focus. I really don't like, for example, doing dishes. However, if I give that activity my full attention, if I make it the most important activity of the moment, I find calmness and peace in the task.

No matter how hard we try, we simply cannot do two things at the same time. Something has to give and all too often someone may suffer. Since we now know that we can do only one thing at a time, doing it mindfully makes it meaningful.

7

EXPECT THE UNEXPECTED

E VEN WITH THE BEST of plans, things happen that we never anticipated. We can't always prepare for them but we should try never to be surprised by them. We've chosen just a few possible unexpected events to share with you in the hopes that you may at least be aware of their possibility.

Road Rage

Road rage is simply something that you want nothing to do with! Nothing good or even close to okay ever comes from it. Law enforcement departments across the country implore us not to acknowledge other drivers' aggressive behavior except perhaps to mouth "sorry" and let them go on their way. If you reply or engage in any contact at all, the whole situation ramps up so fast that before you know it you are screaming at the offending driver and now YOU are full of rage!

A good rule for driving in Los Angeles (and anyplace else for that matter) is to leave early. That should be simple, right? Well, of course, it's not. Parents, persons just entering the work force, students, doctors, lawyers—we all have to deal with life. Getting into the car and getting on our way is the first but not the only challenge. There is so much to do just to get moving. We've got to find our car keys. We've got to buckle up. We've got to start the engine. Then we've got to remember that we forgot something, shut off the engine, un-buckle and go retrieve whatever it is we forgot. Then before we hit the road we've got to gas up because we forgot to do that on our way home last night. It never stops.

We reasonably expect that once we're on the road things will settle down and we'll feel calmer. Regardless of our des-tination, generally someone expects us to arrive on time.

Here's some advice. If you know you are likely to be late, pull off the road and make the call. Taking the time to call is a whole lot better than having someone wonder about your arrival. You'll feel calmer, too.

Sadly, it really doesn't take too much to push us into a road rage state of mind especially if we were feeling frustrated or angry before we even left home. We have to get there and all those other drivers are in our way. The best-case scenario is that it's regular traffic and even though we move slowly we get there. The worst-case scenario is that there's a major in-cident and traffic is stopped for miles! Some of us handle the bad situations better than most. We're already late and then some clown seems to think that the lane we're sitting in is faster than the lane he or she is in and cuts right in front of us with an SUV the size of a garage! Now we're stuck and we can't even see the traffic in front of us.

Sometimes that's all it takes for some drivers to lose it. The results are emotional angst (which as we all know can possi-bly lead to yelling at the kids for no apparent reason when you get home) with sometimes physical and tragically even deadly results. Focusing on something that makes us feel that we're doing all we can to help ourselves through this situation can seriously help us maintain control.

You are in charge of you! This information is quite empowering. It's good for the soul.

Jeff has reported on the aftermath of road rage. He has listened on the scanner as police officers try to stop a person trying to cut off the gravel truck driver who they think is totally responsible for the crack in their windshield! It is not rational behavior.

Shootings sometimes happen because one person cuts off another person on a freeway. Up in the air, Jeff has certainly seen the reactions and results of road rage. Remember the driver who ignored the "Traffic Break" only to be pursued by police and caught? That driver's behavior was a form of road rage. That driver was defying authority. The driver's aggressive behavior disregarded the safety and wellbeing of everyone on that roadway. Jeff has a tough time watching incidents such as these from the air because he's sometimes helpless to do anything to warn or help those in harm's way. Unfortunately it doesn't always end well.

Road rage isn't just a driving phenomenon. The behavior associated with it can happen anyplace and any time. It seems that all living creatures experience and express anger. We humans can learn to control our behavior and express our anger in ways that do no harm. Fundamental to managing our anger is to stop allowing others to push our buttons. We all have those buttons and we all must acquire methods of keeping them in control.

What are some of your buttons? If someone tells you that you're stupid do you fly off the handle? What about if someone cusses you out? What happens then? Can you keep it together if your next-door neighbor while playing with his dog tosses a tennis ball into your yard? What do you do if the person who lives down the hall from you turns the music up too loud? Those might be some of your buttons. It's okay if they aren't but please know that we all have our buttons.

Take a minute to identify a few of your buttons that you don't like having pushed. Now write them down.

....

....

....

....

It's our responsibility to not let anyone push our buttons. That's one way we can keep control of our behavior. Knowing what some of our buttons are helps us expect the unexpected. We don't like people to push our buttons. If we suspect that's about to happen we can make some choices. If we're having a conversation we can change the subject. Or we can ignore the comments of the other person. If we're on the road we can, as law enforcement suggests, ignore the behavior of the other person.

Getting home alive doesn't depend on proving that we're right or responding to every invitation to react. Ignore the one finger salute given you by the driver cutting in front of you. And certainly don't try to catch up and cut in front of the driver who just cut in front of you. It's not about winning. It's about surviving.

We understand that sometimes winning really feels good. On the other hand, a bullet to the chest fired by a gun in the hand of a stranger doesn't feel good at all. Temper is a lousy driver.

If the unthinkable happens and you are stopped and a stranger is coming towards you, lock your doors, stay in your car, and call 911. Then start honking your horn. Human behavior is such that someone will come to your aid while the police are responding.

We don't want to experience road rage in any form. We can minimize the likelihood that we will experience it by knowing our buttons and making sure they don't get pushed. We can ignore the offensive behavior of others. We can remember that safely getting to where we want to be is more important than making our point or winning.

Let the other guy win. That can feel pretty good, too.

Unplanned Stops

Even without a law enforcement traffic break we sometimes need to just stop. And sometimes it's really hard to stop doing what we were doing. Stopping can also take time.

Here are some examples of how long it takes some modes of transportation to stop. These approximations assume a travel speed of 55 miles per hour. A lightweight passenger car, for example, takes about 200 feet to stop if conditions are perfect (tires and brakes are in good condition and the road is dry). A commercial van or bus needs about 230 feet to stop. A commercial truck/trailer rig can stop in about 300 feet. That's about the length of a football field. A light rail train needs about 600 feet to stop—the length of 2 football fields. And the average freight train needs more than a mile or the length of about 18 football fields to stop.

Stopping a vehicle we now see takes time and distance. The amount of time and distance depend on the size of the vehicle and the speed it's traveling. We are urged to keep enough space between our vehicle and the vehicle in front of us to allow for slowing and stopping. We know the danger of trying to cross railroad tracks with a train coming toward us. We also know that sudden stops on the road can be dangerous. We can quickly lose control.

Common wisdom tells us to always be prepared to stop.

We have traffic laws compelling us to keep safe distances between us and the vehicle in front of us, to never go around the railroad crossing barrier or to ignore the flashing lights when a train approaches.

We understand that stopping takes time and distance. For vehicles, that time and distance is determined by speed and vehicle size. For those of us driving our lives and not just our vehicles, we believe that the time and distance required to stop depend on the depth of our commitment to the specific endeavor. Our height and weight don't matter.

Without the traffic breaks of law enforcement, how do we know when to slow down or stop? How do we know when we need to take a deep breath and reset our priorities? We keep in constant touch with our thoughts and our emotions. We listen to our bodies. We utilize our support systems. We daily check our lists of self-care activities. We never forget that we are driving our lives.

We control our routes and our destinations.

8.

BEWARE OF MISSION DRIFT

THIS MIGHT SOUND FAMILIAR. A man decides that his weekend goal is to mow the lawn. (Sorry. I know women also mow the lawns. For the sake of this discussion, though, it was a man.) He gets out the lawn mower. He's using one of those old fashioned, push mowers. He hasn't used it in awhile and immediately notices that the blades are dull. He thinks there's a place nearby that advertised lawn mower blade sharpening and decides to give it a try. He doesn't want to get dead grass on the carpet of the SUV so he goes inside to get some newspapers. The first paper he picks up is yesterday's and he remembers that he hasn't read it yet so he sits down to skim through it before his spouse puts it in the recycling bin. As long as he's reading yesterday's paper he decides to take time for a cup of coffee. He likes milk in his coffee but, even though the coffee is still hot, the milk has gone sour and isn't usable. He decides to quickly run to the store and pick up some milk. He drives the SUV to the store. As long as he's at the store he may as well pick up his dry cleaning because the dry cleaner is close by. The dry cleaner seems to have lost his favorite shirt and, since it's Sunday, he will need a new favorite shirt for Monday so he runs to the mall to select a new shirt.

Okay. I'm sure you see where this is going. By the end of the day, when it's too dark to mow the lawn, the lawn mower is still outside. It hasn't been sharpened or used. The man returns it to the garage and vows to mow next weekend.

That's what mission drift is all about. We drift away from the original mission onto other seemingly important or necessary or even urgent matters. In military parlance this type of distraction is called 'mission creep' because the original objective seems to just slip away incrementally.

This drifting doesn't apply only to weekend chores. We can drift away from life goals too. Accomplishing a mission requires focus. If you want to get to where you want to be on the road and in life, it's essential to keep the destination in mind.

If I want to drive from Los Angeles to San Francisco I may choose to make a few stops or take a few side trips along the way but if my mission is to arrive in San Francisco then I must discipline myself to stay on course. I may stop in Gilroy to buy garlic but once the purchase is made I've got to get back in the car and hit the road. It's possible that along the way I decide that I don't really want to be in San Francisco but let that decision be the result of some serious thinking and not the result of following a distraction.

So what's one of your missions? You can also call them goals if that works better for you. Do you want to learn to tap dance? Do you want to yodel? Do you want to write a book? Do you want to become a nurse? Do you want to grow a garden?

Remember the guy who wanted to mow his lawn? He allowed distractions to keep him from completing that mission.

He drifted away from the original plan. He doubtless could have accomplished grocery and clothing shopping too and still have mowed the lawn and read yesterday's paper.

And what about our drive to San Francisco? What if we get off the 5 and take the 14 and go to Palmdale because we heard about a good restaurant there? Maybe Palmdale could wait for another trip. It's one thing to change our minds about San Francisco. However, if we do change our minds, let's not regret having not driven to San Francisco.

Life is too short and too complicated to regret the decisions we make. However, if we really want to go to San Francisco it is essential that we not allow mission drift to send us off to Palmdale.

Understanding the mission, identifying the goals, helps us get where we want to be on the road and in life.

We hope we've helped you.

FINAL THOUGHTS

9.

Jeff's Pilot Acknowledgments

I started using the term "Airborne Reporter" years ago to clarify to listeners who was doing what from aircraft. Be it television or radio the person on-air was generally thought by the general public and even some in the media, to be at the controls of the aircraft or . . . the pilot. In some cases this is correct however there are different configurations of personnel aboard. In the case of the television broadcast some will use the pilot as the on air talent. The camera operator would be the only other crewmember needed to complete the crew of two. Others in television will use on air talent, camera operator and pilot for a total of three aboard. The other and increasingly popular arrangement in television, is camera operator/on air talent and of course a pilot. With radio it is simply pilot/on air talent as a crew of one or pilot with "Airborne Reporter" for a total of two. The conversation in the electronic news gathering (ENG) airborne world of which is best, most cost effective and safest is an ongoing discussion.

Without the extraordinary skill, commitment and patience of many of the pilots that flew me around for all these years in both helicopters and fixed wing aircraft, my reporting would never have happened. In my case it is without question an example of two thinking as one! The following is a partial list of those I trusted and depended on completely for over 25 years and still would!

Gary Ansell

Gary Suozzi

Wayne Richardson

Kevin LARosa sr.

John Nielson

Aldo Bentivegna

Glen Galbraith

Jonathan Gunn

Dan Benton

Dan Dudek

David G. Gibbs

John Tamburro

Ethan Ruhman

Paul Hollenbeck

Jeff Moir

Scott Bauman

Gary Lineberry

Howard Lewis

Ty Palmer

Adam Bennet

Erin Fitzgerald

Dan Rudert

Vic Hobbs

John Sarviss

Rob Dufau

Lindsay Gow

Bruce Berquist

Craig Dyer

Dale House

David Child

Eric Melton

Estaban Ortiz

Rick Santa Maria

David Spiker

Connor Grey

Adam Ford

Kurt Weikum

Rick Avery

James Shanahan

As of this writing I know I have left a few names out and I sincerely apologize. Please know that you have my utmost respect and will remember you all for the good work you helped me accomplish and a few good laughs. Make that a lot of good laughs!

I want to thank one last pilot. My mother, Peggy, is pictured here with the Luscombe 8A which she flew with skill and confidence. I thank her for all she taught me and for, even to this day, always flying with me.

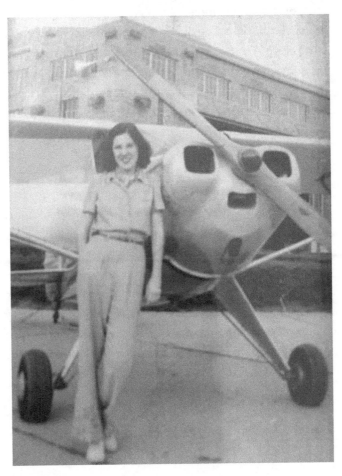

Mary's Newsletter Article

President's Article—Temple Sinai of Glendale

I'm a great fan of Jeff Baugh. On weekday mornings, his voice is generally the first I hear. He sets off my day on a practical and positive note even when all indications are that the day will be gridlocked with complications. Generally his voice also guides me on my sometimes precarious journey back home.

Jeff Baugh is an airborne traffic announcer for radio station KFWB. He appears to fly over the Los Angeles freeways from sunrise to sunset Monday through Friday in a helicopter called Jetcopter 98 saying things like, "The 405 is a mess, take Sepulveda instead," or "Don't get near the 10 West and Grand." He ends his edicts with something along the lines of, "Don't worry. Be patient and we'll get you through this."

Under the best of circumstances, I can barely find my face first thing in the morning. I need Jeff Baugh to guide me and to reassure me that things will eventually work out fine.

I work in Pomona. I live in Glendale. Rarely do I remember much of my daily commute aside from the voices of frenzied newscasters hysterically hyping every minor recent event into epic horror stories of potential if not actual doom and destruction interspersed with the voice of Jeff Baugh assuring me that things will eventually work out okay if I simply heed his advice.

I try to take as many different routes as possible between Glendale and Pomona and Pomona and Glen-

dale. A few weeks ago I decided to take the 10 to the 57 to the 210 to the 134 and thus home. As soon as I had committed myself to the 57, Jeff, in his unflappable and reassuring voice said, "Whatever you do, don't take the 57 north. There is a brush fire where the 57 joins the 210 and traffic is completely stopped. If you are already on the 57, get off at Arrow Highway. Go west until Grand then get back on the 210. You will avoid the fire and the traffic. Just be patient for a little while and we'll get you through this just fine."

I could see the fire in front of me. The 57 was packed and traffic was barely moving. Arrow Highway was two miles away. I knew that if I could just be patient I could get off at Arrow Highway and I would be fine. I worried, though, that everyone else on the 57 was planning on doing the same thing. However, I decided to do exactly as I was told.

Every few seconds Jeff Baugh reminded the hundreds of motorists stuck on the 57 to stay calm, get off on Arrow Highway, and be patient. I stayed in my far right lane ready to compete for the off ramp. The closer I got to Arrow Highway the more astonished I was that I was among the very few cars moving toward that off ramp. The majority of the cars continued in their lanes directly to the fire where the 57 and the 210 merged. This seemed beyond belief to me. Here was old Jeff practically pleading with us to get off at Arrow Highway and there went car after car after car directly toward the brush fire and traffic that clearly was moving nowhere.

I got off at Arrow Highway. I drove west. I turned north on Grand. I got back on the 210 west and continued to Glendale in very light traffic. In back of me the 210 remained closed for several hours right where the 57 joins it.

It must be hard to be Jeff Baugh. His messages are so simple. Take an alternate route. Put a road map in your visor so you can find your own alternate route. Don't be afraid. Be patient. Everything will work out fine. We will get you through this.

Despite his simple prophecies, most people appear to be inordinately committed to maintaining their regular routes. Far better, it seems, to spend hours stuck in traffic than to risk change.

Jeff Baugh's wisdom and this season in our sacred calendar have a lot in common. Every year at this time our tradition urges us to look around us and to change courses if our lives appear to be gridlocked. Our sacred writings and teachings are our roadmaps. Most of us keep them tucked not in our visors for easy reference but lost somewhere amid the unused pages of our Franklin Covey organizers and the instructions to our Palm pilots.

Even when we know change is warranted, it is difficult and scary. The routes are strange and never before traveled. We're not sure they will lead us in the direction we chose even though we seriously question the original choices.

This is the season to change. This is the season to separate ourselves from the multitudes inching imperceptibly but surely toward the brushfire. This is the season to take a different, a safer, a simpler route. This is our season. May we have the courage and the patience to change

And Some Final Acknowledgments

Tracy Dressner proofread this manuscript and helped us out with factual information. Remember that train derailment in Glendale? Tracy is a criminal defense appellate attorney and actually represented the man convicted in that incident on his appeal. Tracy, we thank you so much for all you do for us.

We also thank Jesse Leffer for her cover concept and Pauline Neuwirth not only for designing with passion and heart but for her guidance throughout this project.

And finally we thank Leslie Bergson for her endless proofreading, editing, and correcting. You kept us focused and assured us that we could get to where we wanted to be with this book.

10

NOW HIT THE ROAD
AND LIVE YOUR LIFE

ERE WE ARE AT the end of this particular road. You've read the book. You've made your lists and drawn your maps and created your support crews. You know how to ask for help and you know how important it is to provide help. You've learned from ten significant freeway events how to better manage your life on and off the road. You know the value of having alternate routes and back up plans. You know that it's okay to pull off the road and take a break.

Feel proud of yourself. You've worked hard at this. And be kind to yourself on the road and in life. We are so very proud of you.

It's hard to say goodbye and send you on your way. You stuck with us and we hope we've helped you get to where you want to be on the road and in life.

May your roads be smooth and may you fulfill your mission to live your life knowing peace and contentment.

Drop us a post card from time to time and tell us about your travels. We really do care about you.

Now off you go.